M000206341

Assessment

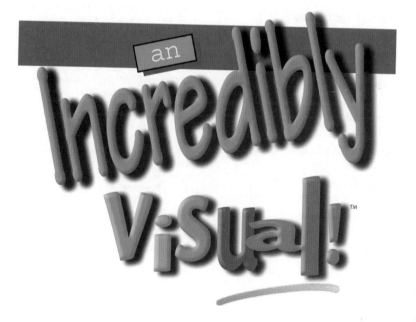

an **Incredibly Visual!**™

Pocket Guide

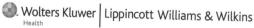
Wolters Kluwer | Lippincott Williams & Wilkins
Health

Philadelphia · Baltimore · New York · London
Buenos Aires · Hong Kong · Sydney · Tokyo

Staff

Executive Publisher
Judith A. Schilling McCann, RN, MSN

Clinical Director
Joan M. Robinson, RN, MSN

Art Director
Elaine Kasmer

Clinical Project Manager
Kate Stout, RN, MSN, CCRN

Editors
Jaime Stockslager Buss, MSPH, ELS; Diane Labus

Illustrator
Bot Roda

Design Assistant
Kate Zulak

Associate Manufacturing Manager
Beth J. Welsh

Editorial Assistants
Karen J. Kirk, Jeri O'Shea, Linda K. Ruhf

Production Manager
Debra Schiff

CONTENTS

Contributors and consultants v

Kim Cooper, RN, MSN
Nursing Department Chair
Ivy Tech Community College
Terre Haute, Ind.

Sally E. Erdel, RN, MS, CNE
Assistant Professor of Nursing
Bethel College
Mishawaka, Ind.

Emilie Fedorov, RN, MSN, ACNS-BC, CNRN
Neuroscience/Surgical Intensive Care Unit Director
St. Mary's Hospital
Madison, Wis.

Cheryl Kabeli, FNP-BC, CNS-BC
Senior Nurse Practitioner
Champlain Valley Cardiothoracic Surgeons
Plattsburgh, N.Y.

Mary Kelly, CRNP, MSN
Nurse Practitioner
Abington (Pa.) Pulmonary & Critical Care Assoc. Ltd.

Priscilla A. Lee, RN, BSN, MSN, NP-C
Nurse Practitioner II
UCLA Gonda Vascular Center
Assistant Clinical Professor
UCLA School of Nursing
Los Angeles

Mary L. Nesbitt, BSN, MAN, CERTIFIED IN-PATIENT OB/GYN
Assistant Professor
William Carey on the Coast
Gulfport, Miss.

Bruce Austin Scott, MSN, ACNS-BC
Nursing Instructor
San Joaquin Delta College
Staff Nurse
Saint Joseph's Medical Center
Stockton, Calif.

Concha Carrillo Sitter, MS, APN, FNP-BC, CGRN
Nurse Practitioner
Sterling Rock Falls Clinic
Sterling, Ill.

Fundamentals

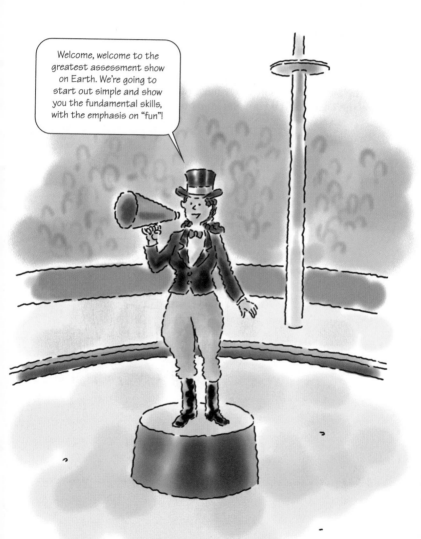

Health history

● Gathers data about the patient and explores past and present problems
  – Biographical data
  – Chief complaint (including specific information about symptoms)
  – Current medications
  – Personal and family medical history
  – Psychological history
  – Functional status
● Subjective data: Information that can be verified only by the patient, such as the patient complaint, "My head hurts."
● Forms the basis for the care plan and holistic treatment approach

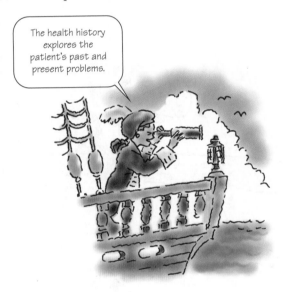

The health history explores the patient's past and present problems.

Evaluating a symptom

Question the patient to identify the symptom bothering him.

⬇

Form a first impression. Does the patient's condition alert you to an emergency?

Yes ⬇   **No** ⬇

Take a brief history to gather more clues.

Take a thorough history to get an overview of the patient's condition. Ask him about associated signs and symptoms.

⬇   ⬇

Perform a focused physical examination to quickly determine the severity of the patient's condition.

Thoroughly examine the patient to evaluate the chief sign or symptom and to detect additional signs and symptoms.

⬇

Evaluate your findings. Are emergency signs or symptoms present?

Yes ⬇   **No** ⬇

Based on your findings, intervene appropriately to stabilize the patient.
Notify the practitioner immediately of the assessment findings and carry out the practitioner's orders.

Evaluate your findings to determine possible causes.

⬇   ⬇

After the patient's condition is stabilized, review your findings to determine possible causes.

Devise an appropriate plan of care.

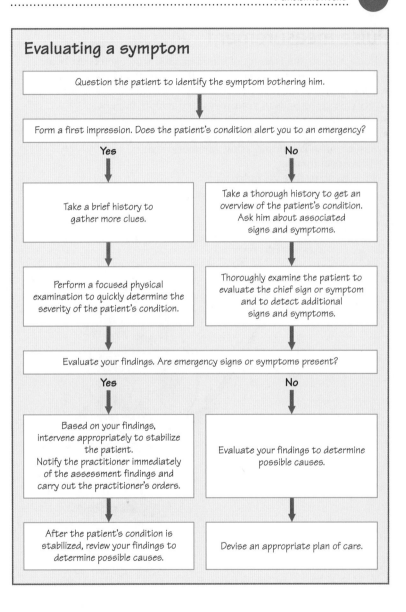

Pulse measurement

- Pulse reflects the amount of blood ejected with each heart beat.
- A normal pulse rate for an adult is between 60 and 100 beats/minute.
- Palpate one of the patient's arterial pulse points (usually the radial artery) using the pads of your index and middle fingers.
- Count the rate for 1 minute (normal or abnormal).
- Assess the rhythm (regular or irregular).
- Assess pulse amplitude using a numeric scale:

  0 = Absent pulse

  +1 = Weak or thready pulse

  +2 = Normal pulse

  +3 = Bounding pulse

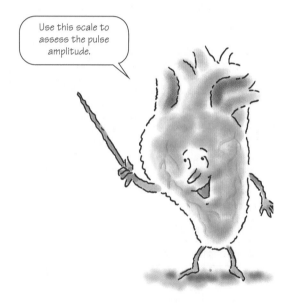

Use this scale to assess the pulse amplitude.

Assessing the pulse rate

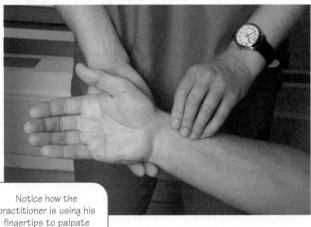

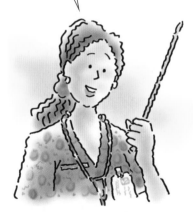

Notice how the practitioner is using his fingertips to palpate the radial pulse.

Blood pressure measurement

- Systolic reading reflects the maximum pressure exerted on the arterial wall at the peak of left ventricular contraction. Normal range is 100 to 119 mm Hg.
- Diastolic reading reflects the minimum pressure exerted on the arterial wall during left ventricular relaxation. Normal diastolic pressure ranges from 60 to 79 mm Hg.
- Use a sphygmomanometer to measure blood pressure.
- Position the patient with his upper arm at heart level and his palm turned up.
- Apply the cuff snugly 1″ (2.5 cm) above the brachial pulse.
- Palpate the brachial or radial pulse with your fingertips while inflating the cuff.
- Inflate the cuff to 30 mm Hg above the point where the pulse disappears.
- Place the diaphragm or bell of the stethoscope over the pulse point.
- Release the valve slowly on the cuff, noting the points where Korotkoff sounds are heard (systolic pressure) and where they disappear (diastolic pressure).

Ensuring accurate blood pressure measurement

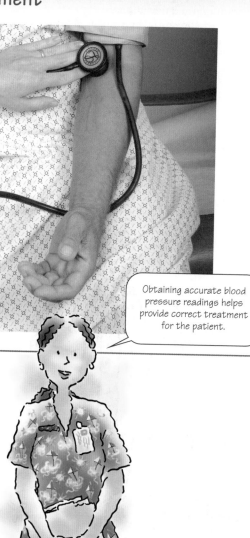

Obtaining accurate blood pressure readings helps provide correct treatment for the patient.

Inspection

● Inspect each body system using vision, smell, and hearing to observe normal conditions and deviations.

● Note color, size, location, movement, texture, symmetry, odors, and sounds as you assess each body part.

● Use inspection to help determine mental status, personality traits, and demeanor by noting appearance and behavioral responses to questions and physical assessment.

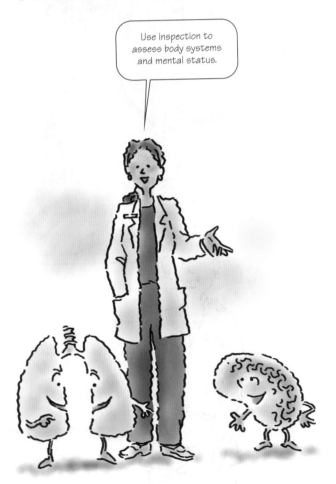

Use inspection to assess body systems and mental status.

Performing inspection

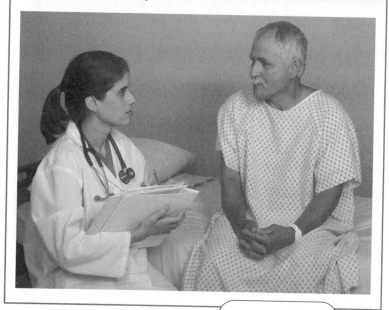

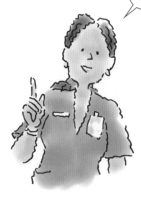

Inspection is about using all of your senses to gather data on the patient.

Palpation

- Palpation requires you to touch the patient with different parts of your hands, using varying degrees of pressure.
- Keep your fingernails short and your hands warm.
- Wear gloves when palpating mucous membranes or areas in contact with body fluids.
- Palpate tender areas last.

Light palpation

- Depress the skin ½″ to ¾″ (1.3 to 1.9 cm) with your finger pads, using the lightest touch possible.
- Assess for texture, tenderness, temperature, moisture, elasticity, pulsations, superficial organs, and masses.

Deep palpation

- Depress the skin 1½″ to 2″ (3.8 to 5 cm) with firm deep pressure. Use one hand on top of the other to exert firmer pressure, if needed.
- Use this technique to feel internal organs and masses for size, shape, tenderness, symmetry, and mobility.

Performing palpation

Light palpation

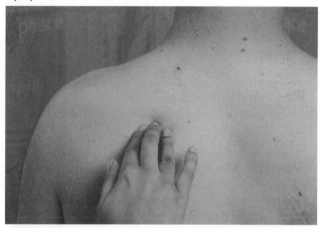

Deep palpation

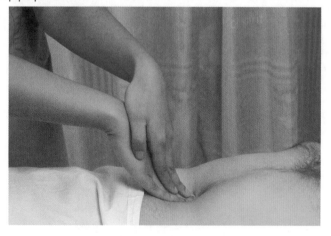

Percussion

● Percussion involves tapping your fingers or hands quickly and sharply against parts of the patient's body to help you locate organ borders; identify organ shape, size, and position; and determine if an organ is solid or filled with fluid or gas.

● Percussion also involves using a trained ear to detect slight variations in sound. Organs and tissues produce sounds of varying loudness, pitch, and duration.

Direct percussion

● Tap directly on the body part using one or two fingers.
● Ask the patient to tell you which areas are painful, and watch for telltale signs of discomfort.

Indirect percussion

● Press the distal part of the middle finger of your nondominant hand firmly on the body part.
● Keep the rest of your hand off the body surface.
● Flex the wrist of your dominant hand and use the middle finger to tap quickly and directly over the point where your other middle finger touches the patient's skin.

See if you can keep this beat. For direct percussion, you tap directly on the body part.

Performing percussion

Direct percussion

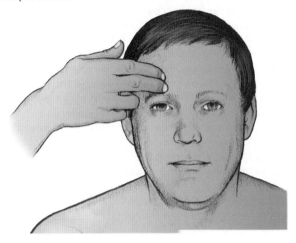

Indirect percussion

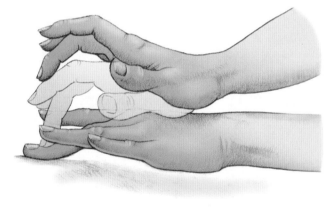

Auscultation

- Auscultation involves listening with a stethoscope for various breath, heart, and bowel sounds.
- Use the diaphragm of the stethoscope to detect high-pitched sounds, such as first (S_1) and second (S_2) heart sounds, bowel sounds, and breath sounds. Hold the diaphragm firmly against the patient's skin, enough to leave a slight ring on the skin afterward.
- Use the bell to pick up low-pitched sounds, such as third (S_3) and fourth (S_4) heart sounds. Hold the bell lightly against the patient's skin, just enough to form a seal. Holding the bell too firmly causes the skin to act as a diaphragm, obliterating low-pitched sounds.
- Listen to and try to identify the characteristics of one sound at a time.
- Be sure to provide a quiet environment.
- Expose the area to be auscultated, because bed linens and clothing can interfere with sounds.
- Warm the stethoscope head before applying it to the skin.
- Close your eyes to help focus your attention.

Performing auscultation

Using the diaphragm

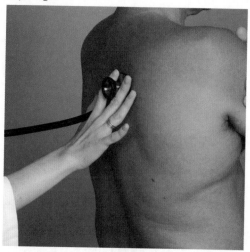

Using the bell

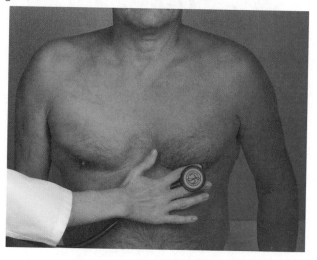

Documentation

● Document history and physical assessment information according to facility policy.

● Utilize documentation forms provided by the facility and provide as much information as possible.

● Document general information about the patient, including the patient's age, race, sex, general appearance, height, weight, body mass, vital signs, communication skills, behavior, awareness, orientation, and level of cooperation.

● Precisely record all information obtained using the four assessment techniques.

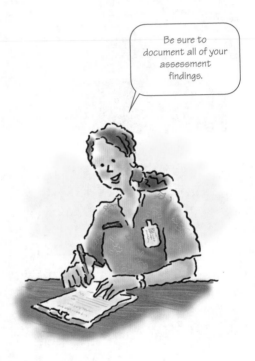

Recording initial assessment findings

General information

Name __Henry Gibson__

Age __55__   Sex __M__   Height __163 cm__   Weight __57 kg__

T __37° C__   P __76__   R __14__   B/P __(R) 150/90 sitting (L) 148/88 sitting__

Room __328__

Admission time __0800__

Admission date __1-28-08__

Doctor __Manzel__

Admitting diagnosis __Pneumonia__

_____

_____

_____

_____

_____

Patient's stated reason for hospitalization __"To get rid of the pneumonia"__

Allergies __Penicillin__
__Codeine__

Current medications __None__

Drug	Dosage	Last taken

General survey

In no acute distress, slender, appears younger than stated age.
Alert and well-groomed. Communicates well. Makes eye contact and
expresses appropriate concern throughout exam.— _C. Smith, RN_

_____

_____

2

Skin, hair, and nails

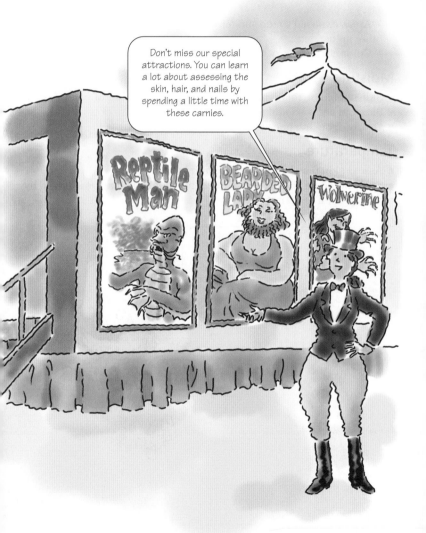

Don't miss our special attractions. You can learn a lot about assessing the skin, hair, and nails by spending a little time with these carnies.

Skin assessment

- Observe the skin's overall appearance.
- Inspect and palpate the skin area by area, focusing on color, moisture, temperature, texture, and turgor.

Color

- Look for areas of bruising, cyanosis, pallor, and erythema.
- Check for uniformity of color and hypopigmented or hyperpigmented areas.
  - Areas exposed to the sun may show darker pigmentation than other areas.
  - Color changes vary depending on skin pigmentation.

Moisture

- Skin should be relativity dry, with a minimal amount of perspiration.
- Skinfold areas should also be fairly dry.
- Overly dry skin appears red and flaky.

Temperature

- Assess skin temperature for warmth or coolness.
- Skin should be slightly warm or slightly cool and may be affected by environmental temperature.

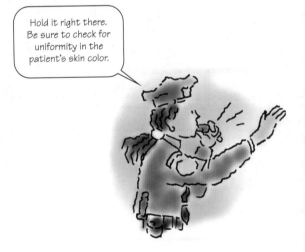

(Text continues on page 22.)

Assessing skin color and moisture

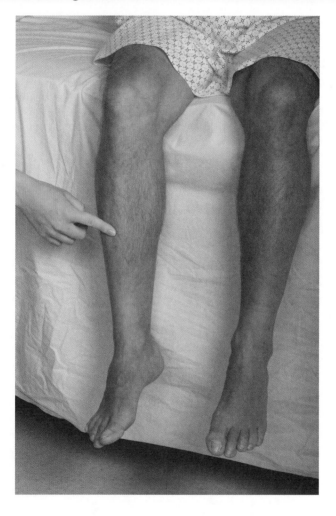

Skin assessment (continued)

Texture

● Inspect and palpate the skin's texture, noting its thickness and mobility. It should look smooth and be intact.

Turgor

● Palpate the skin to evaluate the patient's hydration status.
● To evaluate skin turgor, gently squeeze the skin on the forearm or sternal area between your thumb and forefinger.
  – If the skin quickly returns to its original shape, the patient has normal turgor.
  – If the skin returns slowly over 30 seconds or maintains a tented position (as shown), the skin has poor turgor.

Palpating the skin can tell a lot about your patient's hydration status . . . Gulp . . . Feeling a little thirsty, myself!

Assessing skin turgor

Squeezing the skin

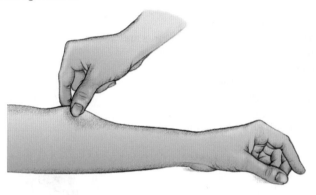

Evaluating return to original shape

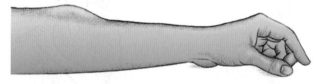

Lesions

- Classify the lesion as primary (new) or secondary (a change in a primary lesion):
  - Primary lesions include bullae, cysts, macules, nodules, papules, pustules, vesicles, and wheals.
  - Secondary lesions include fissures and ulcers.
- Determine if the lesion is solid or fluid-filled.
- Describe its characteristics, pattern, location, and distribution, including a description of symmetry, borders, color, shape, configuration, diameter, and drainage.

A penlight can help you determine whether a lesion is solid or fluid-filled.

Memory jogger

To remember what to assess when evaluating a lesion, think of the first five letters of the alphabet:

Asymmetry

Border

Color and **C**onfiguration

Diameter and **D**rainage

Evolution (progression) of lesion.

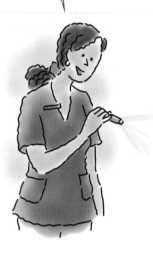

Identifying primary lesions

Bulla
A large, fluid-filled blister that's usually 1 cm or more in diameter

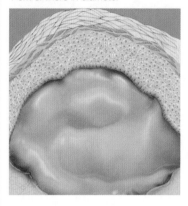

Cyst
A closed sac in or under the skin that contains fluid or semisolid material

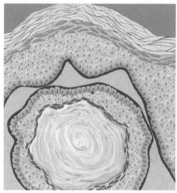

Macule
A small, discolored spot or patch on the skin

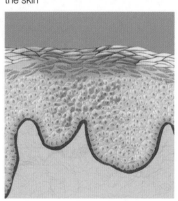

Nodule
A raised lesion detectable by touch that's usually 1 cm or more in diameter

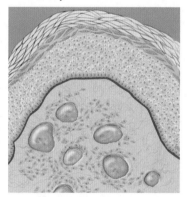

(continued)

Identifying primary lesions *(continued)*

Papule
A solid, raised lesion that's usually less than 1 cm in diameter

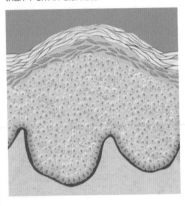

Pustule
A small, pus-filled lesion

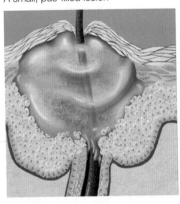

Vesicle
A circumscribed, raised lesion that contains serous fluid and is usually less than 1 cm in diameter

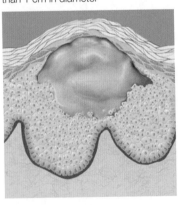

Wheal
A raised, reddish area that's commonly itchy and lasts 24 hours or less

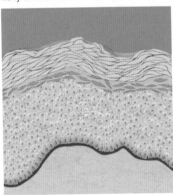

Identifying secondary lesions

Fissure
A painful, cracklike lesion of skin that extends at least into the dermis

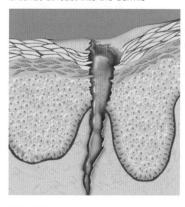

Ulcer
A craterlike lesion of the skin that usually extends at least into the dermis

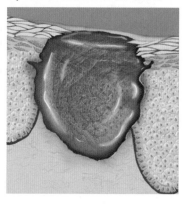

Lesion characteristics

- Examine the lesion to see if it looks the same on both sides and check the borders.
- Notice configuration patterns, because many skin diseases have typical patterns.
- Assess lesion distribution:
  - Generalized: distributed all over the body
  - Regionalized: limited to one area of the body
  - Localized: sharply limited to a specific area
  - Scattered: dispersed either densely or widely
  - Intertriginous: limited to areas where skin comes in contact with itself.

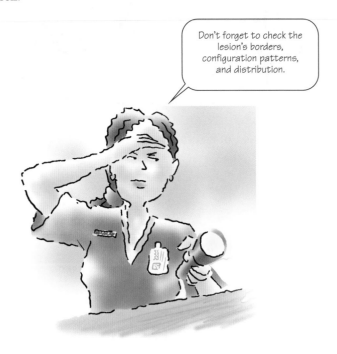

Don't forget to check the lesion's borders, configuration patterns, and distribution.

Recognizing lesion shapes and configurations

Lesion shapes

Discoid
Round or oval

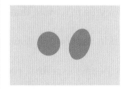

Annular
Circular with central clearing

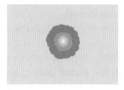

Target (bull's eye)
Annular with central internal activity

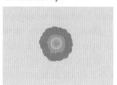

Lesion configurations

Discrete
Individual lesions are separate and distinct.

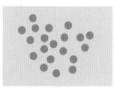

Grouped
Lesions are clustered together.

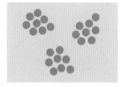

Confluent
Lesions merge so that discrete lesions aren't visible or palpable.

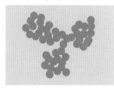

Dermatomal
Lesions form a line or an arch and follow a dermatome.

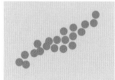

Carcinomas

- Lesions may be benign, such as a benign nevus or mole. However, changes in an existing growth on the skin or a new growth that ulcerates or doesn't heal could indicate cancer or a precancerous lesion.
- Types of skin cancer:
    - Precancerous actinic keratosis: abnormal change in keratinocytes that can become squamous cell carcinoma
    - Dysplastic nevus: abnormal growth of melanocytes in a mole that can become malignant melanoma
    - Basal cell carcinoma: most common type of skin cancer that usually spreads only locally
    - Squamous cell carcinoma: type of cancer that begins as a firm, red nodule or scaly, crusted, flat lesion and can spread if not treated
    - Malignant melanoma: type of cancer that can arise on normal skin or from an existing mole and can spread to other areas of skin, lymph nodes, or internal organs, if not promptly treated

Identifying skin cancer

Precancerous actinic keratosis

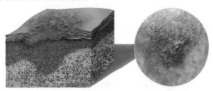

Dysplastic nevus

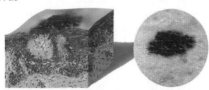

Basal cell carcinoma

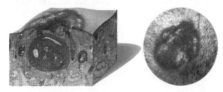

Squamous cell carcinoma

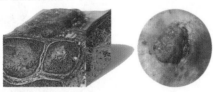

Malignant melanoma

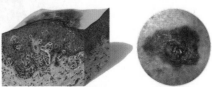

Pressure ulcers

- Pressure ulcers are localized areas of skin breakdown that occur as a result of prolonged pressure or pressure combined with friction or shear.
- Necrotic tissue develops as a result of diminished vascular supply to the area.
- Staging of pressure ulcers reflects the anatomic depth of affected tissue:
  - Suspected deep tissue injury: purple or reddened area of intact skin
  - Stage I: nonblanchable area of redness
  - Stage II: open or closed blister; shallow open area with red wound bed (partial thickness loss); slough not present
  - Stage III: open area with subcutaneous fat possibly present (full thickness loss); slough may be present; tunneling or undermining may be present
  - Stage IV: open area with muscle, bone, or tendon exposed (full thickness loss)
  - Unstageable: open area with full thickness loss; slough or eschar covering wound bed

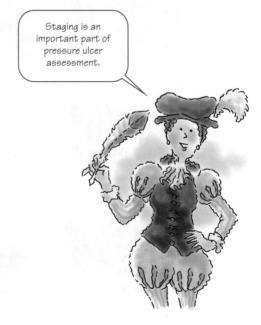

Staging is an important part of pressure ulcer assessment.

Staging pressure ulcers

Stage I

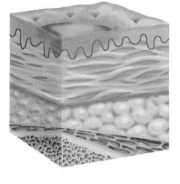

Stage II

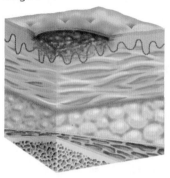

Stage III

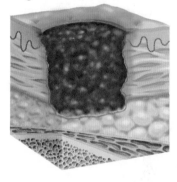

Stage IV

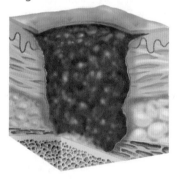

Suspected deep tissue injury

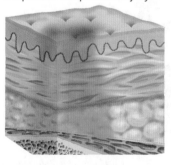

Unstageable

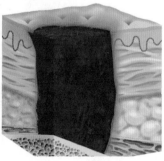

Other skin abnormalities

Psoriasis

- Psoriasis is a chronic disease of marked epidermal thickening.
- Plaques are symmetrical and generally appear as red bases topped with silvery scales.
- Lesions most commonly occur on the scalp, elbows, and knees.

Contact dermatitis

- Contact dermatitis is an inflammatory disorder that results from contact with an irritant.
- Primary lesions include vesicles; large, oozing bullae; and red macules that appear at localized areas of redness.
- Lesions may itch and burn.

Urticaria

- Urticaria is an allergic reaction that appears suddenly as pink, edematous papules or wheals.
- Lesions may become large and contain vesicles.

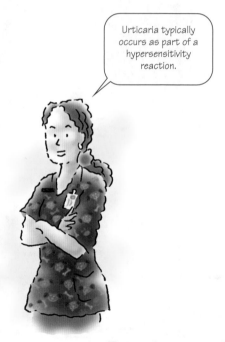

Urticaria typically occurs as part of a hypersensitivity reaction.

(Text continues on page 36.)

Identifying psoriasis, contact dermatitis, and urticaria

Psoriasis

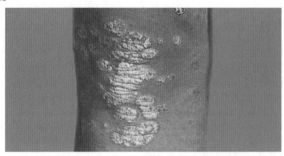

Contact dermatitis

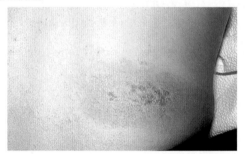

Urticaria (hives)

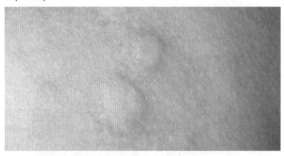

Other skin abnormalities (continued)

Herpes zoster

● Infection appears as a group of vesicles or crusted lesions along a nerve root.
● Vesicles are usually unilateral and appear mostly on the trunk.
● Lesions cause pain but not a rash.

Scabies

● Mites, which can be picked up from an infested person, burrow under the skin and cause scabies lesions.
● Lesions appear in a straight or zigzagging line that's about ⅜″ (1 cm) long, with a black dot at the end.
● Scabies lesions are commonly seen between the fingers, at the bends of the elbows and knees, and around the groin and abdomen.
● Lesions itch and may cause a rash.

Tinea corporis (ringworm)

● Characterized by round, red, scaly lesions that are accompanied by intense itching.
● Individual rings of lesions may connect to form patches with scalloped edges.

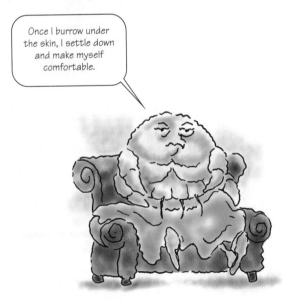

Identifying herpes zoster, scabies, and tinea corporis

Herpes zoster

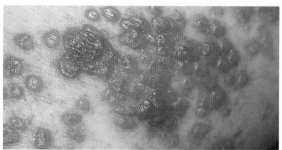

Scabies

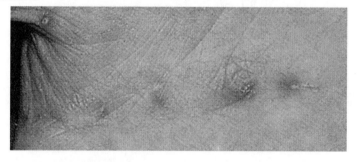

Tinea corporis (ringworm)

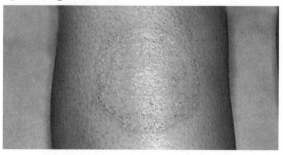

Hair assessment

- Inspect and palpate the hair over the patient's entire body.
- Note the distribution, quantity, texture, and color. The quantity and distribution of head and body hair vary among patients. However, hair should be evenly distributed over the entire body.
- Check for patterns of hair loss and growth.
- Examine the scalp for erythema, scaling, and encrustation.
- Excessive hair loss with scalp crusting may indicate ringworm infestation.

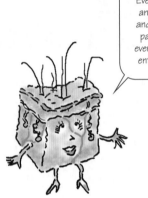

Even though the quantity and distribution of head and body hair vary among patients, hair should be evenly distributed over the entire body. Check it out!

Looking at hair growth

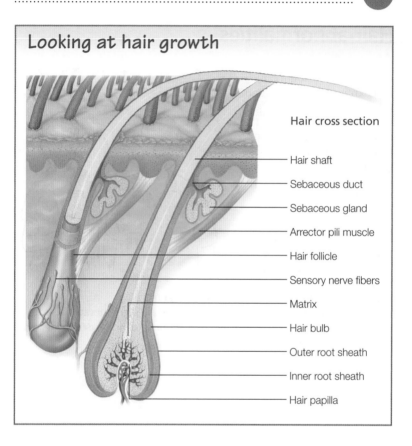

Hair cross section

- Hair shaft
- Sebaceous duct
- Sebaceous gland
- Arrector pili muscle
- Hair follicle
- Sensory nerve fibers
- Matrix
- Hair bulb
- Outer root sheath
- Inner root sheath
- Hair papilla

Hair abnormalities

Alopecia

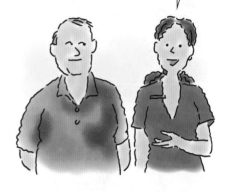

Alopecia is more common in men.

● Occurs more commonly and extensively in men than in women
● May be a normal part of aging or may occur as a result of pyrogenic infections, chemical trauma, ingestion of certain drugs, endocrinopathy, and other disorders

Hirsutism

● Excessive hairiness in women that develops on the body and face
● Localized hirsutism may occur on pigmented nevi
● Generalized hirsutism can result from certain drug therapy or from endocrine problems, such as Cushing's syndrome, polycystic ovary syndrome, and acromegaly

Identifying alopecia and hirsutism

Alopecia

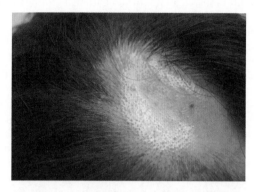

Hirsutism

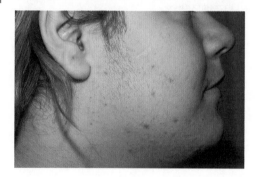

Nail assessment

- Appearance of nails can be a critical indicator of systemic illness.
- Overall condition tells a lot about the patient's grooming habits and ability to provide self-care.
- Examine the color of the nails:
    - Light-skinned people have pinkish nails.
    - Dark-skinned people have brown nails.
    - Brown pigmented bands in the nail beds are normal in dark-skinned people and abnormal in light-skinned people.
    - Smokers' nails may be yellow as a result of nicotine stains.
- Inspect the shape and contour of the nails. The surface of the nail should be either slightly curved or flat.
- Palpate the nail bed to check the thickness of the nail and the strength of its attachment to the bed.
- Press on the nail bed to assess peripheral circulation. Note how long the color takes to return when you release the nail bed. Color should return in less than 3 seconds.

Looking at the nail

Nail cross section

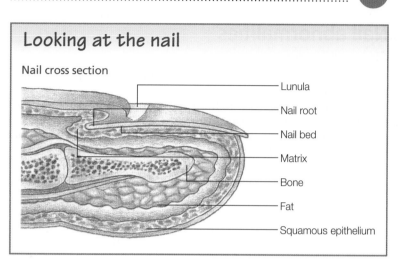

- Lunula
- Nail root
- Nail bed
- Matrix
- Bone
- Fat
- Squamous epithelium

Nail abnormalities

Clubbed fingers

● To assess for clubbing, check the angle of the nail base; it's normally about 160 degrees.

● An elevated proximal edge of the nail that produces an angle greater than 180 degrees suggests clubbing.

● A clubbed nail is also thickened and curved at the end, and the distal phalanx looks rounder and wider than normal.

(Text continues on page 46.)

Evaluating clubbed fingers

Normal finger

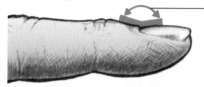

Normal angle (160 degrees)

Clubbed finger

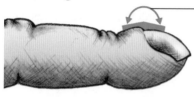

Angle greater than 180 degrees

> The nails on clubbed fingers are commonly enlarged and curved.

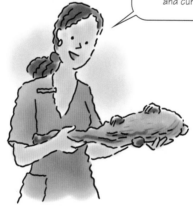

Nail abnormalities *(continued)*

Splinter hemorrhages

- Reddish brown, narrow streaks under the nails that run in the same direction as nail growth
- Caused by minor trauma, but can also occur in patients with bacterial endocarditis

Terry's nails

- Transverse bands of white that cover the nail
- Absent lunula
- Can affect one or all nail beds
- Associated with aging and chronic disorders, such as cirrhosis, heart failure, and type 2 diabetes

Identifying splinter hemorrhages and Terry's nails

Splinter hemorrhages

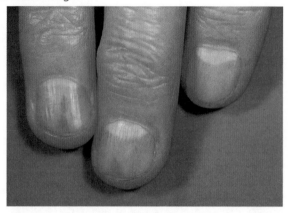

Terry's nails

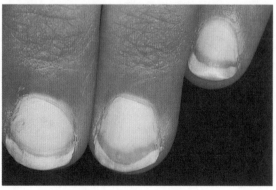

3
Eyes and ears

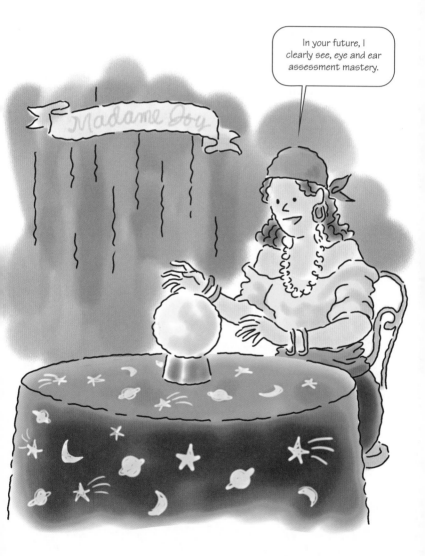

External eye assessment

● Inspect the eyes, starting at the scalp line, and determine if they're in a normal position (about one-third of the way down the face and about one eye's width apart from each other).

● Examine the eyelids, which should cover the top quarter of the iris so the eyes look alike; eyes should open and close completely; lid margins should be pink and eyelashes should turn outward.

● Look at the irises, which should appear flat and be the same size, color, and shape.

● Examine the corneas, which should be clear, have no lesions, and appear convex.

● Examine the corneas by shining a penlight in the eye, first from each side and then from straight ahead.

● Test corneal sensitivity by lightly touching the cornea with a wisp of cotton.

Assessing corneal sensitivity

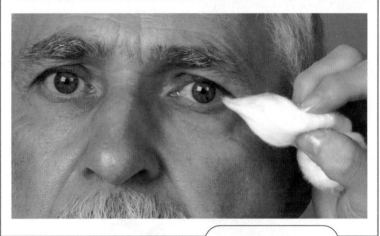

Remember that contact lens wearers may have reduced corneal sensitivity because they're used to having foreign objects in their eyes.

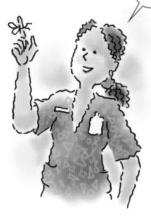

Conjunctiva assessment

- Inspect the bulbar conjunctiva:
  - Ask the patient to look up.
  - Gently pull the lower eyelid down.
  - The conjunctiva should be clear and shiny.
  - Note excessive redness or exudate.
- Assess the sclera. It should be white or buff.

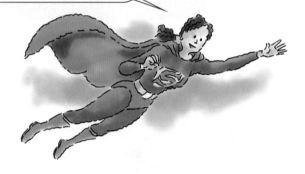

Inspecting the conjunctiva and sclera

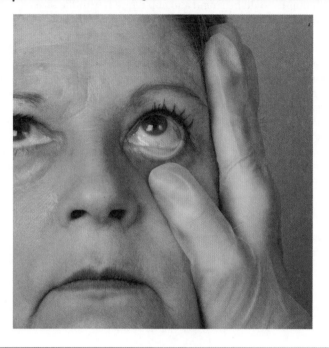

Pupil assessment

- Each pupil should be round and about one-fourth the size of the iris in normal room light. The pupils should be equal in size.
- Test each pupil for direct and consensual response:
    – In a slightly darkened room, hold a penlight about 20″ (50 cm) from the patient's eyes and direct the light at the eye from the side.
    – Note the reaction of the pupil you're testing (direct) and the opposite pupil (consensual); both should react the same way.
- Test accommodation:
    – Place your finger about 4″ (10 cm) from the bridge of the patient's nose.
    – Ask him to look at a fixed object in the distance and then look at your finger; his pupils should constrict and his eyes should converge as he focuses on your finger.

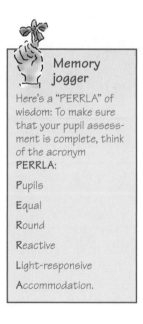

Memory jogger

Here's a "PERRLA" of wisdom: To make sure that your pupil assessment is complete, think of the acronym **PERRLA**:

Pupils

Equal

Round

Reactive

Light-responsive

Accommodation.

Grading pupil size

1 mm   2 mm   3 mm   4 mm   5 mm   6 mm   7 mm   8 mm   9 mm

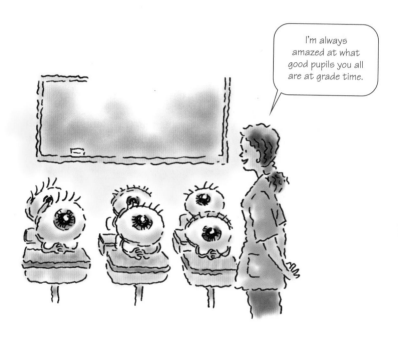

Eye muscle function assessment

Corneal light reflex

- Ask the patient to look straight ahead, and shine a penlight on the bridge of his nose from 12″ to 15″ (30.5 to 38 cm) away.
- The light should fall at the same spot on each cornea. If it doesn't, the eyes aren't being held in the same plane by the extraocular muscles.

Cardinal positions of gaze

- This test evaluates the function of the oculomotor, trigeminal, and abducens cranial nerves and the extraocular muscles.
- Hold a pencil or other small object directly in front of the patient's nose at a distance of about 18″ (45 cm).
- Ask the patient to follow the object with his eyes without moving his head.
- Move the object to each of the six cardinal positions, returning to the midpoint after each movement.
- Note abnormal findings, such as nystagmus (involuntary, rhythmic oscillation of the eyeballs) or amblyopia (failure of one eye to follow an object).

Evaluating cardinal positions of gaze

Right superior (RS)

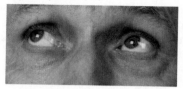

Left superior (LS)

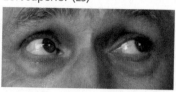

Right lateral (RL)

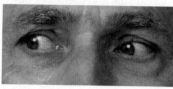

Left lateral (LL)

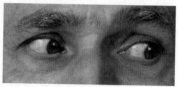

Right inferior (RI)

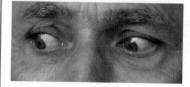

Left inferior (LI)

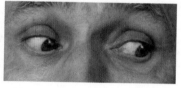

Internal eye assessment

- Use an ophthalmoscope to perform direct observation of the eye's internal structures.
- Adjust the lens dial to see the internal structures. Use the green, positive numbers on the disc to focus on near objects, such as the patient's cornea or lens. Use the red, minus numbers to focus on distant objects, such as the retina.
- Before beginning your examination, ask the patient to remove his contact lenses or eyeglasses.
- Darken the room to dilate the pupils.
- Ask the patient to focus on a point behind you, and use the ophthalmoscope to elicit the red reflex and examine the anterior chamber, lens, retina, and optic disc.

Looking at the retina

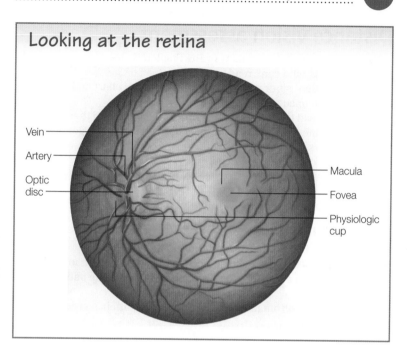

Vein

Artery

Optic disc

Macula

Fovea

Physiologic cup

Distance vision assessment

- Use the Snellen alphabet chart or the Snellen E chart (for young children or patients who can't read).
- Have the patient sit or stand 20′ (6.1 m) from the chart and cover his left eye with an opaque object.
- Ask him to read the letters on one line of the chart and then to move downward to increasingly smaller lines until he can no longer discern all of the letters.
- Repeat the test on the other eye.
- If the patient wears corrective lenses, have him repeat the test wearing them.
- Record the results with and without correction.

Recording results

- Visual acuity is recorded as a fraction.
- The top number (20) is the distance between the patient and the chart. The bottom number is the distance from which the patient can read the chart.
- The larger the bottom number, the poorer the patient's vision.

Snellen charts

Snellen alphabet chart

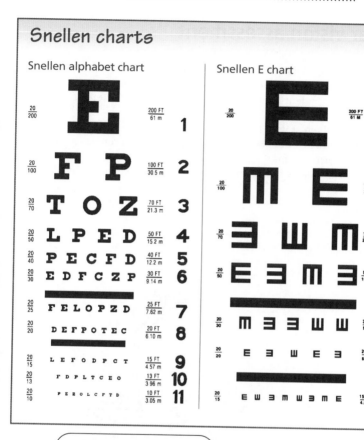

$\frac{20}{200}$	**E**	$\frac{200\ FT}{61\ m}$ **1**
$\frac{20}{100}$	**F P**	$\frac{100\ FT}{30.5\ m}$ **2**
$\frac{20}{70}$	**T O Z**	$\frac{70\ FT}{21.3\ m}$ **3**
$\frac{20}{50}$	**L P E D**	$\frac{50\ FT}{15.2\ m}$ **4**
$\frac{20}{40}$	**P E C F D**	$\frac{40\ FT}{12.2\ m}$ **5**
$\frac{20}{30}$	**E D F C Z P**	$\frac{30\ FT}{9.14\ m}$ **6**
$\frac{20}{25}$	**F E L O P Z D**	$\frac{25\ FT}{7.62\ m}$ **7**
$\frac{20}{20}$	**D E F P O T E C**	$\frac{20\ FT}{6.10\ m}$ **8**
$\frac{20}{15}$	L E F O D P C T	$\frac{15\ FT}{4.57\ m}$ **9**
$\frac{20}{13}$	F D P L T C E O	$\frac{13\ FT}{3.96\ m}$ **10**
$\frac{20}{10}$	P E Z O L C F T D	$\frac{10\ FT}{3.05\ m}$ **11**

Snellen E chart

$\frac{20}{200}$		$\frac{200\ FT}{61\ M}$
$\frac{20}{100}$		$\frac{100\ FT}{30.5\ M}$
$\frac{20}{70}$		$\frac{70\ FT}{21.7\ M}$
$\frac{20}{50}$		$\frac{50\ FT}{15.2\ M}$
$\frac{20}{30}$		$\frac{30\ FT}{9.1\ M}$
$\frac{20}{20}$		$\frac{20\ FT}{6.1\ M}$
$\frac{20}{15}$		$\frac{15\ FT}{4.6\ M}$

Does your patient wear contacts or glasses? Remember to test his vision with and without his corrective lenses.

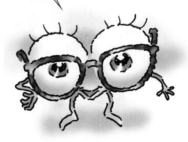

Near vision assessment

● Use the Rosenbaum card to evaluate near vision:
  – Cover one of the patient's eyes with an opaque object.
  – Hold the Rosenbaum card 14″ (35.5 cm) from the eyes.
  – Have the patient read the line with the smallest letters he can distinguish.
  – Repeat the test with the other eye.
  – If the patient wears corrective lenses, have him repeat the test while wearing them.
  – Record visual accommodation with and without corrective lenses.

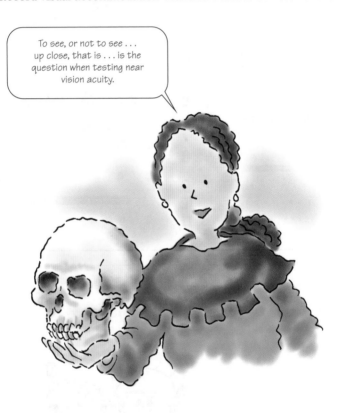

To see, or not to see . . . up close, that is . . . is the question when testing near vision acuity.

Rosenbaum card

	distance equivalent
95	$\frac{20}{800}$

ACCOMMODATION TEST

	Point	Jaeger	
874			$\frac{20}{400}$
2843	26	16	$\frac{20}{200}$
638 ЕШƎ XOO	14	10	$\frac{20}{100}$
8745 ƎП Ш OXO	10	7	$\frac{20}{70}$
63925 ПЕƎ XOX	8	5	$\frac{20}{50}$
428365 ШЕП oxo	6	3	$\frac{20}{40}$
374258 ƎШƎ xxo	5	2	$\frac{20}{30}$
93·826 ■■■ xoo	4	1	$\frac{20}{25}$
······· ■■■ ···	3	1+	$\frac{20}{20}$

Card is held in good light 14 inches from eye. Record vision for each eye separately with and without glasses. Presbyopic patients should read through bifocal segment. Check myopes with glasses only.

DESIGN COURTESY J. G. ROSENBAUM M.D. CLEVELAND OHIO

PUPIL GAUGE (mm.)

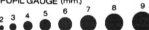

2 3 4 5 6 7 8 9

Eye abnormalities

Conjunctivitis

- Characterized by hyperemia of the conjunctiva with predominate redness in the eye periphery
- Usually begins in one eye and rapidly spreads by contamination to the other eye
- Accompanied by mild discomfort
- Doesn't affect vision except for some blurring caused by watery or mucopurulent eye discharge

Periorbital edema

- Swelling around the eye
- May result from allergies, local inflammation, fluid-retaining disorders, or crying

Ptosis

- Drooping upper eyelid
- May be caused by an interruption in sympathetic innervations to the eyelid, muscle weakness, or damage to the oculomotor nerve

(Text continues on page 66.)

Identifying external eye abnormalities

Conjunctivitis

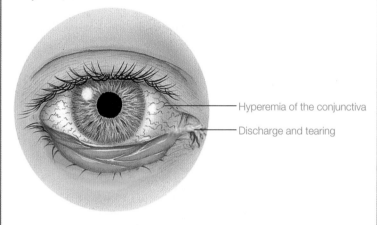

Hyperemia of the conjunctiva

Discharge and tearing

Periorbital edema

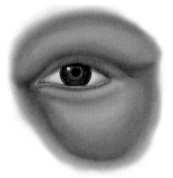

Ptosis

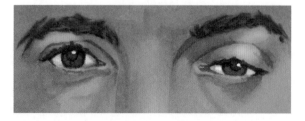

Eye abnormalities *(continued)*

Acute angle-closure glaucoma

- Characterized by a rapid onset of unilateral inflammation, eye pain and pressure, and photophobia
- Causes decreased vision, moderate pupil dilation, nonreactive pupillary response, and clouding of the cornea
- Results in changes in the retinal vessels and enlargement of the physiologic cup, which can be found on ophthalmoscopic examination

Cataract

- Opacity of the lens or lens capsule
- Develops gradually
- Causes vision loss

Macular degeneration

- Atrophy of the macular disk
- Causes irreversible central vision loss
- Age-related type: results from the formation of drusen or subretinal neovascular membrane changes in the macular region

Identifying internal eye abnormalities

Acute angle-closure glaucoma

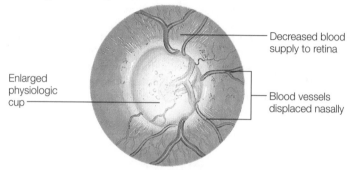

Enlarged physiologic cup

Decreased blood supply to retina

Blood vessels displaced nasally

Cataract

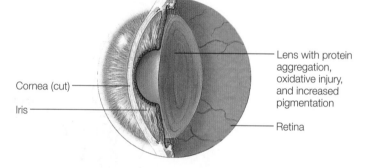

Cornea (cut)

Iris

Lens with protein aggregation, oxidative injury, and increased pigmentation

Retina

Macular degeneration

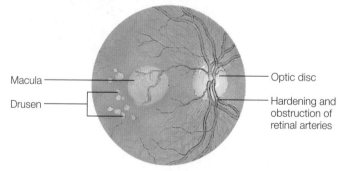

Macula

Drusen

Optic disc

Hardening and obstruction of retinal arteries

External ear inspection

● Observe the ears for position and symmetry. The top of each ear should line up with the outer corner of the eye, and the ears should look symmetrical, with an angle of attachment of no more than 10 degrees.

● Inspect the auricle for lesions, drainage, and redness. Pull the helix back and note if it's tender. Inspect and palpate the mastoid area behind each auricle, noting tenderness, redness, or warmth.

● Inspect the opening of the ear canal, noting discharge, redness, odor, or the presence of nodules or cysts. Note that patients have varying amounts of hair and cerumen (earwax) in the ear canal.

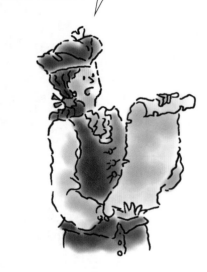

Hear ye, hear ye! Be sure to inspect the patient's ears for position and symmetry.

Looking at the external ear

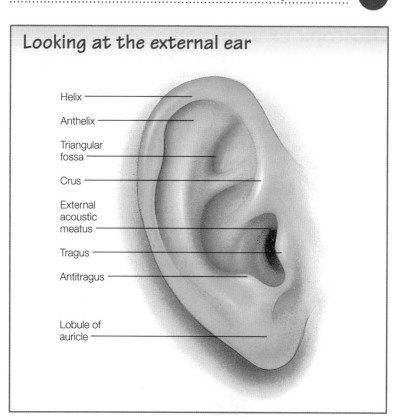

Helix

Anthelix

Triangular
fossa

Crus

External
acoustic
meatus

Tragus

Antitragus

Lobule of
auricle

Otoscopic examination

● Examine the auditory canal, tympanic membrane, and malleus.

● Check the canal for foreign bodies and discharge before inserting the speculum into the patient's ear.

● Palpate the tragus (the cartilaginous projection anterior to the external opening of the ear) and pull the auricle up. If the patient reports tenderness, don't insert the speculum. The patient might have otitis externa, and inserting the speculum could be painful.

● After inserting the speculum, rotate it for a complete view of the tympanic membrane

   – The membrane should appear pearl gray, glistening, and transparent.

   – The annulus should be white and denser than the rest of the membrane.

   – Look for a light reflex; if it is displaced or absent, the tympanic membrane may be bulging, inflamed, or retracted.

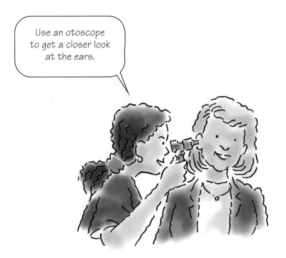

Examining the inner ear

Positioning the ear canal

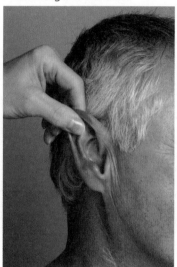

Positioning the otoscope

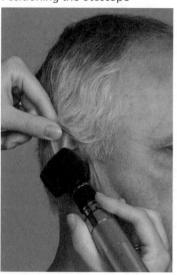

Viewing the structures

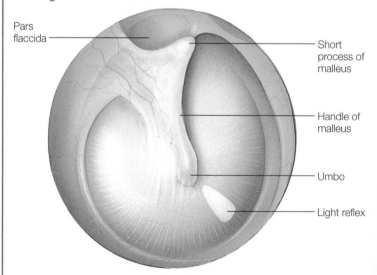

Pars flaccida

Short process of malleus

Handle of malleus

Umbo

Light reflex

Weber's test

- Perform Weber's test to evaluate bone conduction (you'll use a tuning fork that's tuned to the frequency of normal speech [512 cycles/second]).
- To perform the test:
  - Lightly strike the tuning fork against your hand.
  - Place the vibrating fork on the patient's forehead at the midline or on top of his head.

Results	Description
Normal	Patient hears tone equally well in both ears.
Right or left lateralization	Patient hears tone better in one ear.
Conductive hearing loss	Patient hears tone only in his impaired ear.
Sensorineural hearing loss	Patient hears tone only in his unaffected ear.

Performing Weber's test

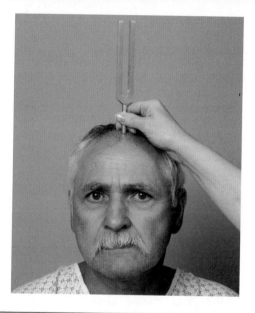

Rinne test

- Perform the Rinne test to compare air conduction (AC) of sound with bone conduction (BC) of sound.
- To perform the test:
  - Strike the tuning fork against your hand.
  - Place the vibrating fork over the patient's mastoid process.
  - Ask the patient to tell you when the tone stops; note the time in seconds.
  - Move the still-vibrating tuning fork to the ear's opening, without touching the ear.
  - Ask the patient to tell you when the tone stops; note the time in seconds.

Results	Description
Normal hearing	Patient hears AC tone twice as long as he hears BC tone (AC > BC).
Conductive hearing loss	Patient hears BC tone as long as or longer than he hears AC tone (BC ≥ AC).
Sensorineural hearing loss	Patient hears AC tone longer than he hears BC tone (AC > BC).

Performing the Rinne test

Placing tuning fork over the mastoid process

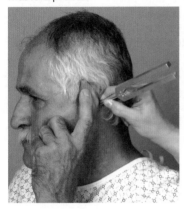

Placing tuning fork near ear's opening

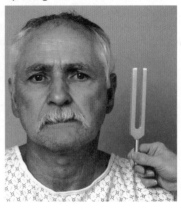

Otitis media

- Inflammation of the middle ear that results from disruption of eustachian tube patency
- Usually has a rapid onset and a short duration
- Infected fluid may collect in the middle ear
- May be accompanied by severe, deep, throbbing pain; conductive hearing loss; mild to high fever; tinnitus; dizziness; nausea and vomiting

Looking at acute otitis media

Otoscopic view

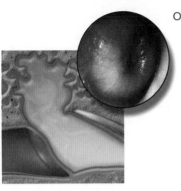

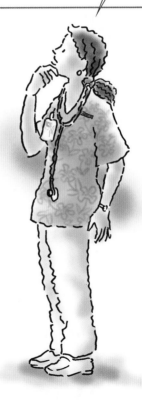

Otitis media can be acute or chronic, suppurative or secretory.

Complications of otitis media

Otitis media with effusion

- Characterized by fluid in the middle ear
- May not cause symptoms
- May be acute, subacute, or chronic

Cholesteatoma

- Abnormal skin growth or epithelial cyst in the middle ear
- Usually results from repeated infections

Perforation

- Hole in the tympanic membrane
- Caused by trauma or chronic negative pressure in the middle ear

Assessing complications of otitis media

Otitis media with effusion

Cholesteatoma

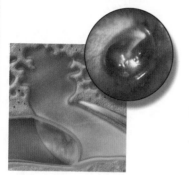

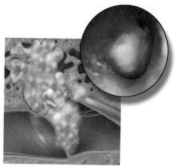

Perforation

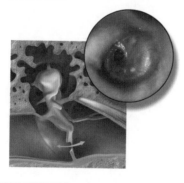

4

Nose, mouth, throat, and neck

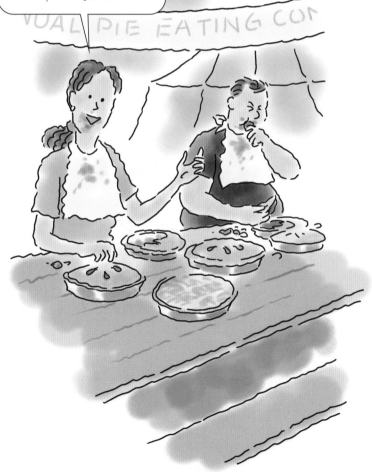

Nose inspection

● Observe the patient's nose for position, symmetry, and color. Note variations, such as discoloration, swelling, and deformity. Variations in size and shape are primarily caused by differences in cartilage and the amount of fibroadipose tissue.

● Observe for nasal discharge and flaring of the nostrils:
  – If discharge is present, note the color, quantity, and consistency.
  – If flaring is present, observe for other signs of respiratory distress.

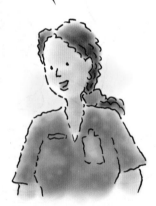

Everybody "nose" that the nose is more than just the sensory organ of smell. It also plays a key role in the respiratory system.

Looking at nasopharyngeal structures

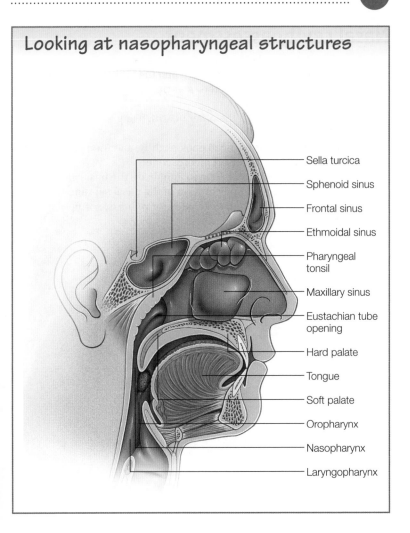

- Sella turcica
- Sphenoid sinus
- Frontal sinus
- Ethmoidal sinus
- Pharyngeal tonsil
- Maxillary sinus
- Eustachian tube opening
- Hard palate
- Tongue
- Soft palate
- Oropharynx
- Nasopharynx
- Laryngopharynx

Nasal cavity assessment

- Test nasal patency and olfactory nerve (cranial nerve I) function:
  - Ask the patient to block one nostril and then inhale a familiar aromatic substance through the other nostril.
  - Ask him to identify the odor.
  - Repeat the process with the other nostril, using a different aroma.
- Inspect the nasal cavity:
  - Ask the patient to tilt his head back slightly, and then push up the tip of his nose and gently insert an otoscope.
  - Use the light from the otoscope to illuminate the nasal cavities.
  - Check for deviation and perforation of the nasal septum.
  - Examine the vestibule and turbinates for redness, softness, swelling, and discharge.

Inspecting the nasal cavity

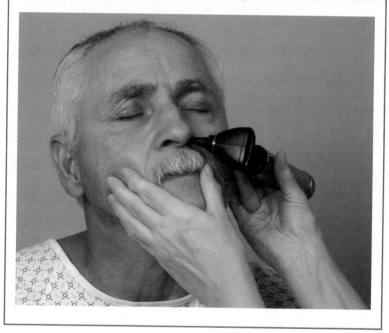

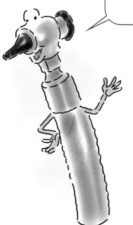

Let me shed some light on your assessment.

Nostril assessment

● Examine the nostrils using a nasal speculum, a penlight or small flashlight, or an otoscope with a short, wide attachment:
  – Have the patient sit in front of you, with his head tilted back.
  – Insert the tip of the speculum into one nostril to the point where the blade widens.
  – Slowly open the speculum as wide as possible without causing discomfort.
  – Shine the flashlight into the nostril to illuminate the area.
  – Observe the color and patency of the nostril and check for exudate.
  – Repeat with the other nostril.
● Palpate the patient's nose with your thumb and forefinger, assessing for pain, tenderness, swelling, and deformity.

Inspecting the nostrils

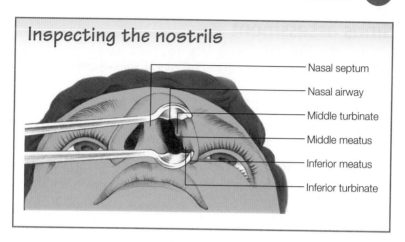

- Nasal septum
- Nasal airway
- Middle turbinate
- Middle meatus
- Inferior meatus
- Inferior turbinate

Sinus assessment

● Palpate the sinuses. Remember, only the frontal and maxillary sinuses are accessible; the ethmoidal and sphenoidal sinuses cannot be palpated.

Frontal sinuses

● Check for swelling around the eyes, especially over the sinus areas.
● Palpate the frontal and maxillary sinuses, checking for tenderness.

Maxillary sinuses

● Gently press your thumbs on each side of the nose, just below the cheekbones.

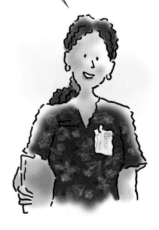

If the frontal and maxillary sinuses are infected, you can assume that the other sinuses are as well.

Palpating the maxillary sinuses

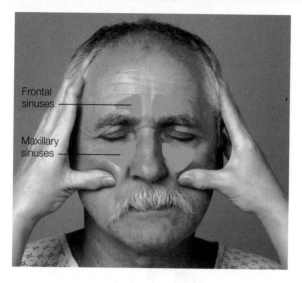

Frontal sinuses

Maxillary sinuses

Transillumination of the sinuses

● Use transillumination to detect fluid or pus in the sinuses as well as tumors and obstructions.
● Darken the room.
● For the frontal sinuses, place the penlight on the supraorbital ring and direct the light upward.
● For the maxillary sinuses, place the penlight on the patient's cheekbone just below the eye and ask the patient to open her mouth.

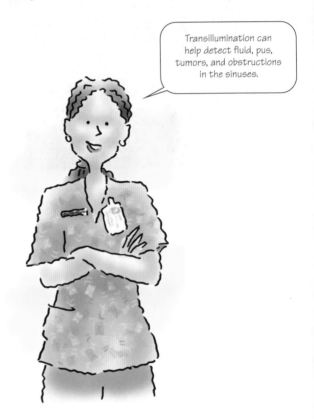

Transillumination can help detect fluid, pus, tumors, and obstructions in the sinuses.

Transilluminating the sinuses

Frontal sinus

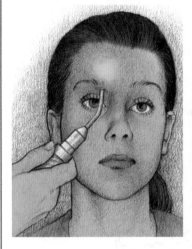

Maxillary sinus

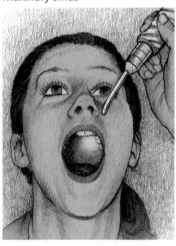

Nose abnormalities

● Obstruction of the nasal mucous membranes accompanied by a thin mucous discharge may indicate systemic disorders; nasal or sinus disorders, such as a deviated septum; trauma, such as a basilar skull fracture; excessive use of vasoconstricting nose drops or sprays; and allergy or exposure to irritants, such as dust, tobacco smoke, and fumes.

● Nasal drainage accompanied by sinus tenderness and fever may suggest acute sinusitis.

● Thick white, yellow, or greenish drainage may suggest infection.

● Clear, thin drainage may indicate rhinitis or may be cerebrospinal fluid leaking from a basilar skull fracture.

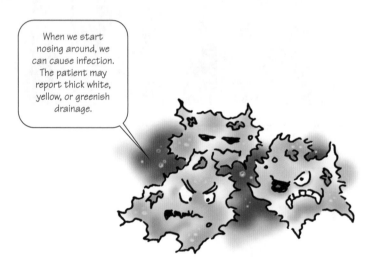

Identifying other nasal symptoms

Symptom	Key facts	Possible causes
Epistaxis	• Refers to nosebleed	• Coagulation disorders • Trauma • Other hematologic disorders • Renal disorders
Flaring	• Refers to dilation that occurs during inspiration • Normal to some extent during quiet breathing but marked regular flaring is abnormal	• Respiratory distress
Stuffiness and discharge	• Refers to obstruction of the nasal mucous membranes accompanied by secretions	• Common cold • Sinusitis • Trauma • Allergies • Exposure to irritants • Deviated septum

Mouth assessment

- Inspect the patient's lips.
- Put on gloves and palpate the lips for bumps and surface abnormalities.
- Instruct the patient to open his mouth, and then place a tongue blade on his tongue.
- Observe the gingivae (gums).
- Inspect the teeth. Note their condition and any absent teeth.
- If the patient is wearing dentures, note the fit; then inspect the gums underneath them.
- Ask the patient to raise the tip of her tongue and touch the palate directly behind the front teeth.
- Inspect the ventral surface of the tongue and the floor of the mouth. Wrap a piece of gauze around the tip of the tongue and move the tongue first to one side and then the other to inspect the lateral borders.
- Expect these normal findings:
  - Lips: pink, moist, and symmetrical; a bluish hue or flecked pigmentation may occur in dark-skinned patients
  - Oral mucosa: pink, smooth, and moist; increased pigmentation may occur in dark-skinned patients
  - Gingivae: pink and moist, with clearly defined margins at each tooth

Inspecting the tongue

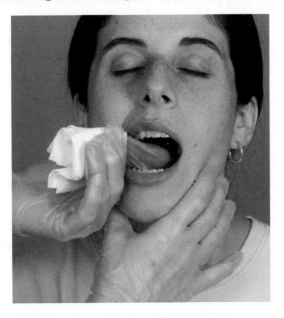

Mouth abnormalities

Herpes simplex (type 1)

- Recurrent viral infection caused by human herpesvirus
- Characterized by initial brief period of prodromal tingling and itching, followed by primary lesion eruption as vesicles on an erythematous base
- Characterized later by ruptured vesicles that leave a painful ulcer, followed by a yellow crust

Angioedema

- Commonly associated with an allergic reaction
- Develops rapidly
- Presents subcutaneously or dermally and produces nonpitting, nonpruritic swelling of subcutaneous tissue and deep wheals, usually on the lips, hands, feet, eyelids, or genitalia

Leukoplakia

- Painless, white patches that may appear on the tongue or the mucous membranes of the mouth
- Considered precancerous lesions

Candidiasis

- Characterized by cream-colored or white patches on the tongue, mouth, or pharynx
- Caused by the organism *Candida albicans* in most cases

Identifying herpes simplex, angioedema, leukoplakia, and candidiasis

Herpes simplex (type 1)

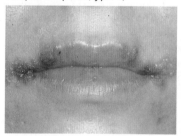

Angioedema

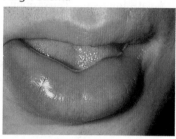

Leukoplakia

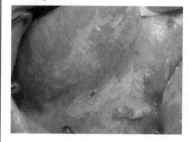

Candidiasis

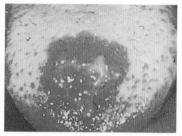

Throat assessment

- Inspect the oropharynx by shining a penlight on the uvula and palate.
- Insert a tongue blade into the mouth to depress the tongue.
- Ask the patient to say "Ahhh" while observing for movement of the soft palate and uvula. The oropharynx and uvula should be pink and moist, without inflammation or exudate. The tonsils should be pink and moist, without hypertrophy.
- Assess the patient's gag reflex by gently touching the back of the pharynx with a cotton-tipped applicator or the tongue blade. This action should produce a bilateral response.

Inspecting the oropharynx

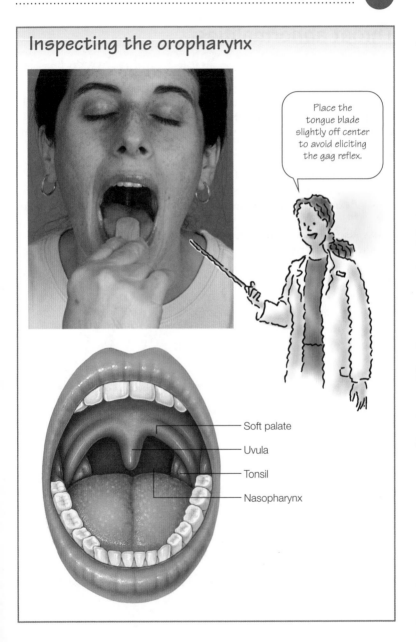

Place the tongue blade slightly off center to avoid eliciting the gag reflex.

Soft palate
Uvula
Tonsil
Nasopharynx

Throat abnormalities

Tonsillitis

- Usually begins with a mild to severe sore throat
- May also produce dysphagia, fever, swelling and tenderness of the lymph nodes, and redness in the throat
- With exudative tonsillitis, a white exudate appears on the tonsils

Pharyngitis

- Acute or chronic inflammation of the pharynx
- Produces a sore throat and slight difficulty swallowing
- Usually caused by a virus, such as a rhinovirus, coronavirus, or adenovirus
- May also be caused by a bacterial infection, such as from group A beta-hemolytic streptococci

Identifying tonsillitis and pharyngitis

Tonsillitis

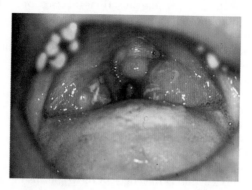

Pharyngitis

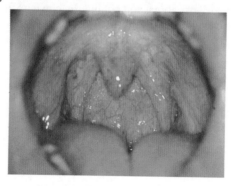

Neck assessment

● Observe the patient's neck. It should be symmetrical, and the skin should be taut. Note scars, visible pulsations, masses, or swelling.

● Ask the patient to move his neck through the entire range of motion and to shrug his shoulders.

● Using the finger pads of both hands, bilaterally palpate the chain of lymph nodes in the following sequence:

  – Periauricular: in front of the ear
  – Postauricular: behind the ear, superficial to the mastoid process
  – Occipital: at the base of the skull
  – Tonsillar: at the angle of the mandible
  – Submandibular: between the angle and the tip of the mandible
  – Submental: behind the tip of the mandible
  – Superficial cervical: superficially along the sternomastoid muscle
  – Posterior cervical: along the edges of the trapezius muscle
  – Deep, anterior cervical: deep under the sternomastoid muscle
  – Supraclavicular: just above and behind the clavicle, in the angle formed by the clavicle and the sternomastoid muscle

Palpating the lymph nodes

Preauricular

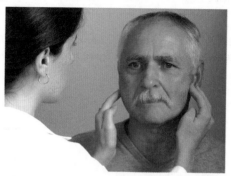

Submandibular

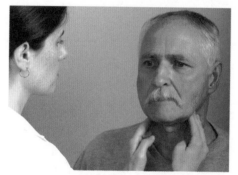

Supraclavicular

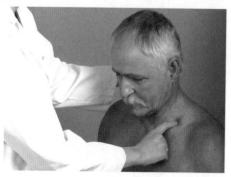

Thyroid palpation

- Stand behind the patient and put your hands around his neck, with the fingers of both hands over the lower trachea.
- Ask him to swallow as you feel the thyroid isthmus, which should rise with swallowing.
- Displace the thyroid to the right and then to the left, palpating both lobes for enlargement, nodules, tenderness, or a gritty sensation.

Palpating the thyroid

Palpating the thyroid

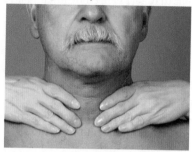

Normal thyroid on swallowing

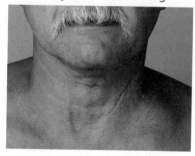

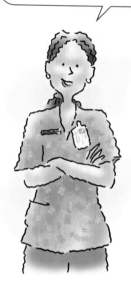

Lowering the patient's chin slightly and turning it toward the side you're palpating can help relax the muscle and facilitate assessment.

Thyroid abnormalities

Simple (nontoxic) goiter

- Involves thyroid gland enlargement that isn't caused by inflammation or a neoplasm
- Commonly classified as endemic or sporadic
- Enlargement can range from a mildly enlarged gland to a massive multinodular goiter

Graves' disease (toxic goiter)

- Most common form of thyrotoxicosis
- Characterized by such classic features as enlarged thyroid, nervousness, heat intolerance, weight loss, sweating, frequent bowel movements, tremor, palpations, and exophthalmos

Toxic multinodular goiter

- Commonly occurs in the elderly
- Form of thyrotoxicosis that involves overproduction of thyroid hormone by one or more autonomously functioning nodules within a diffusely enlarged gland
- Characterized by several palpable nodes

Identifying goiter

Simple (nontoxic) goiter

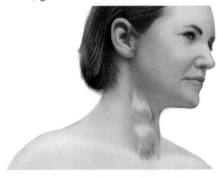

Graves' disease (toxic goiter)

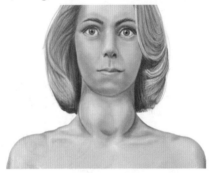

Toxic multinodular goiter

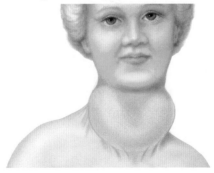

Trachea palpation

- Place your finger along one side of the trachea.
- Assess the distance between the trachea's outer edge and the sternocleidomastoid muscle.
- Assess the distance on the other side and compare the two distances—they should be the same.
- If the trachea isn't midline, possible causes include:
  - atelectasis
  - thyroid enlargement
  - pleural effusion
  - tumor
  - pneumothorax.

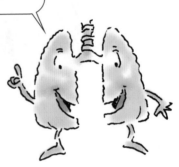

Palpating the trachea

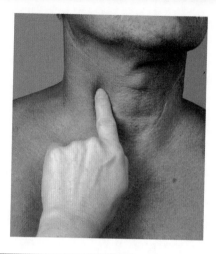

5

Neurologic system

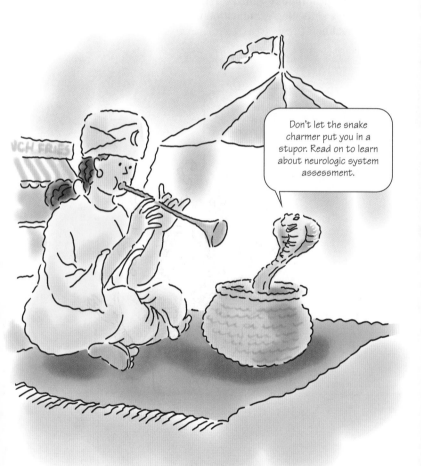

Don't let the snake charmer put you in a stupor. Read on to learn about neurologic system assessment.

Mental status assessment

- Mental status assessment begins when you talk with a patient during the health history.
- Talking with a patient helps you assess:
  - orientation
  - level of consciousness (LOC)
  - ability to formulate and produce speech.
- Be sure to ask questions that require more than "yes" or "no" answers; otherwise, confusion might not be immediately apparent.
- Observe the patient's appearance and behavior.
- Note inappropriate responses to the situation and conversation.
- Perform a screening examination if you have doubts about a patient's mental health.

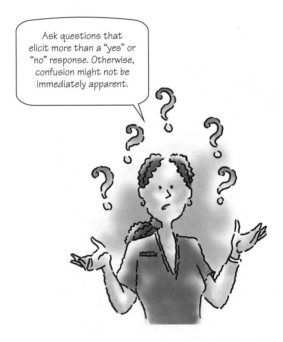

Ask questions that elicit more than a "yes" or "no" response. Otherwise, confusion might not be immediately apparent.

Performing a quick check of mental status

Question	Function screened
What's your name?	Orientation to person
What's your mother's name?	Orientation to other people
What year is it?	Orientation to time
Where are you now?	Orientation to place
How old are you?	Memory
Where were you born?	Remote memory
What did you have for breakfast?	Recent memory
Who's currently the U.S. president?	General knowledge
Can you count backward from 20 to 1?	Attention span and calculation skills

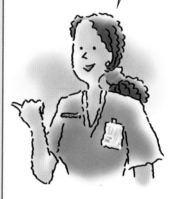

An incorrect answer to one of these quick-check questions might mean that you'll need to perform a full mental status examination.

Level of consciousness

● Clearly describe the patient's response to various stimuli using these terms:
  – Alert—follows commands and responds appropriately to stimuli
  – Lethargic—is drowsy or has delayed response to stimuli
  – Stuporous—requires vigorous stimulation for a response
  – Comatose—has no response to verbal or painful stimuli.
● Use the Glasgow Coma Scale to objectively assess the patient's LOC:
  – Rate the patient's responses according to the scale; then add the scores for the best response in each category to achieve the total score.
  – A total score of less than 9 indicates severe brain injury.

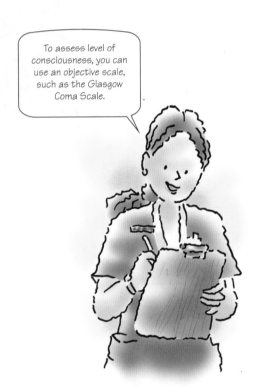

To assess level of consciousness, you can use an objective scale, such as the Glasgow Coma Scale.

Using the Glasgow Coma Scale

Test	Score	Patient's response
Eye opening		
Spontaneously	4	Opens eyes spontaneously
To speech	3	Opens eyes to verbal command
To pain	2	Opens eyes to painful stimulus
None	1	Doesn't open eyes in response to stimulus
Motor response		
Obeys	6	Reacts to verbal command
Localizes	5	Identifies localized pain
Withdraws	4	Flexes and withdraws from painful stimulus
Abnormal flexion	3	Assumes a decorticate position
Abnormal extension	2	Assumes a decerebrate position
None	1	No response; lies flaccid
Verbal response		
Oriented	5	Is oriented and converses
Confused	4	Is disoriented and confused
Inappropriate words	3	Replies randomly with incorrect words
Incomprehensible	2	Moans or screams
None	1	No response

Cranial nerve assessment

● Cranial nerves (CNs) transmit motor messages, sensory messages, or both, primarily between the brain and brain stem and between the head and neck.

● CN assessment reveals valuable information about the condition of the central nervous system.

● Some CNs are more vulnerable to the effects of increased intracranial pressure (ICP).

● Initial assessment focuses on four key nerves:
  – CN II: Optic
  – CN III: Oculomotor
  – CN IV: Trochlear
  – CN VI: Abducens

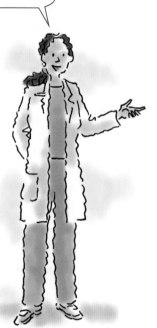

To remember which nerve goes with which function, memorize this silly sentence. Can you find the four "key" nerves on the next page?

Memory jogger

Use the following mnemonic to remember which cranial nerves have sensory functions (S), motor functions (M), or both (B):

I: **S**ome

II: **S**ay

III: **M**arry

IV: **M**oney

V: **B**ut

VI: **M**y

VII: **B**rother

VIII: **S**ays

IX: **B**ad

X: **B**usiness

XI: **M**arries

XII: **M**oney

(Text continues on page 118.)

Identifying the cranial nerves

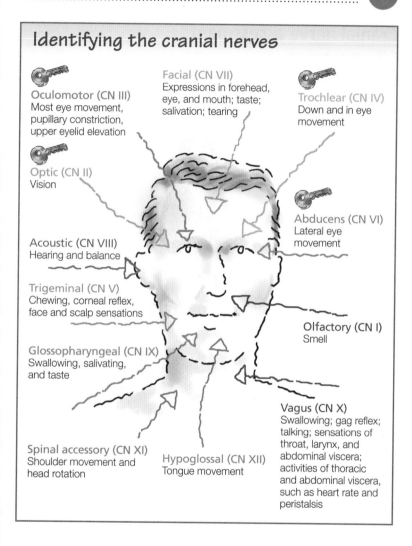

Oculomotor (CN III)
Most eye movement, pupillary constriction, upper eyelid elevation

Optic (CN II)
Vision

Facial (CN VII)
Expressions in forehead, eye, and mouth; taste; salivation; tearing

Trochlear (CN IV)
Down and in eye movement

Abducens (CN VI)
Lateral eye movement

Acoustic (CN VIII)
Hearing and balance

Trigeminal (CN V)
Chewing, corneal reflex, face and scalp sensations

Glossopharyngeal (CN IX)
Swallowing, salivating, and taste

Olfactory (CN I)
Smell

Spinal accessory (CN XI)
Shoulder movement and head rotation

Hypoglossal (CN XII)
Tongue movement

Vagus (CN X)
Swallowing; gag reflex; talking; sensations of throat, larynx, and abdominal viscera; activities of thoracic and abdominal viscera, such as heart rate and peristalsis

Cranial nerve assessment *(continued)*

Olfactory nerve

- Make sure the patient's nostrils are patent.
- Ask the patient to close her eyes, and then occlude one nostril.
- Ask the patient to identify at least two common scented substances, such as coffee and soap.
- Repeat for the other nostril.

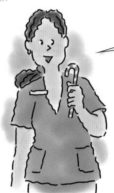

Avoid using stringent scents, such as peppermint, to test the olfactory nerve, because these scents can stimulate the trigeminal nerve.

Optic nerve

- Test the patient's visual acuity quickly and informally by having him read a newspaper. You can formally evaluate visual acuity with a Snellen chart and Rosenbaum card (see pages 60 to 63).
- Test the patient's visual fields using confrontation.
- Examine the fundus of the optic nerve (see page 59).

(Text continues on page 120.)

Testing the olfactory nerve

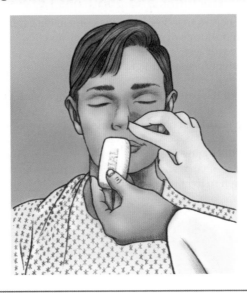

Cranial nerve assessment *(continued)*
Oculomotor, trochlear, and abducens nerves

- Assess these nerves together using the corneal light reflex test and the six cardinal positions of gaze (see pages 56 and 57).
- Perform the cover test:
  - Ask the patient to stare straight ahead and focus on a distant object.
  - Cover one of the patient's eyes with an opaque card. Observe eye movement.
  - Remove the card and observe the previously covered eye for any movement.
  - Repeat on the opposite eye.
- Inspect the size, shape, and symmetry of the pupils as well as the pupillary reaction to light (see page 55).

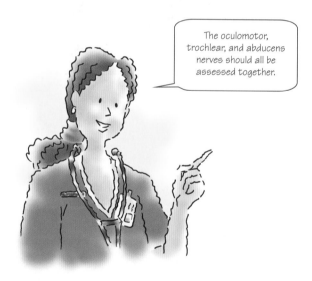

The oculomotor, trochlear, and abducens nerves should all be assessed together.

(Text continues on page 122.)

Performing the cover test

Covering the eye

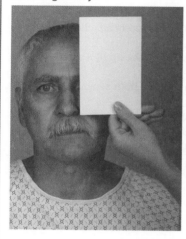

Uncovering the eye

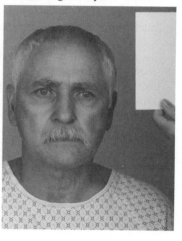

Cranial nerve assessment (continued)

Trigeminal nerve

- Assess the sensory component:
  - Ask the patient to close his eyes.
  - Touch him with a wisp of cotton on his forehead, cheek, and jaw on each side.
  - Test pain perception by gently touching the tip of a safety pin to the same three areas.
  - Ask the patient to describe and compare both sensations.
- Test the motor component:
  - Ask the patient to clench his teeth.
  - Palpate the temporal and masseter muscles, noting their strength.
- Test the corneal reflex by touching a wisp of cotton to the cornea (see page 51); blinking is the normal response.

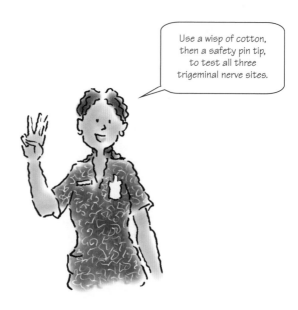

Use a wisp of cotton, then a safety pin tip, to test all three trigeminal nerve sites.

(Text continues on page 124.)

Identifying trigeminal nerve assessment sites

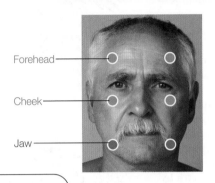

Forehead

Cheek

Jaw

Ask the patient to compare the sensations he feels. If the trigeminal nerve is doing its job, the patient should be able to differentiate soft from sharp.

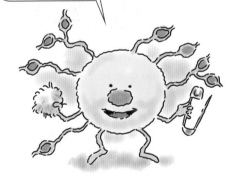

Cranial nerve assessment *(continued)*

Facial nerve

- Test sensory function by placing items with various tastes—for example, sugar (sweet), salt, and lemon juice (sour)—on the anterior portion of the patient's tongue.
- Assess motor function by observing the patient's face for symmetry at rest and when he smiles, frowns, and raises his eyebrows.
- Test muscle strength by instructing the patient to tightly close both eyes and then attempting to open his eyes.

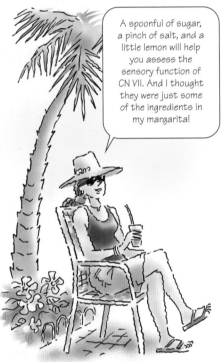

A spoonful of sugar, a pinch of salt, and a little lemon will help you assess the sensory function of CN VII. And I thought they were just some of the ingredients in my margarita!

Acoustic nerve

- To assess acoustic nerve function, perform Weber's test and the Rinne test (see pages 72 to 75).

Glossopharyngeal and vagus nerves

- Test these nerves together because their innervations overlap in the pharynx.
- Listen to the patient's voice.
- Check the gag reflex:
  - Touch the tip of a tongue blade against the posterior pharynx and then ask the patient to open wide and say "ah."
- Watch for symmetrical, upward movement of the soft palate and uvula.
- Check that the uvula is in a midline position.

(Text continues on page 126.)

Testing motor function of the facial nerve

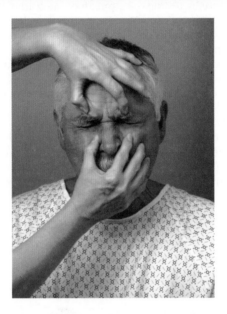

Cranial nerve assessment (continued)

Spinal accessory nerve

● Assess this nerve by testing the strength of the sternocleidomastoid muscles and the upper portion of the trapezius muscle:
   – Place your palm against the patient's cheek, and ask him to turn his head as you apply resistance.
   – Place your hand on the patient's shoulder, and ask him to shrug as you apply resistance.
   – Repeat the tests on the other side, and compare the results.

Hypoglossal nerve

● Assess this nerve by observing the patient's tongue. The tongue should be symmetrical and in a midline position, without tremors or fasciculations.
● Test tongue strength by asking the patient to push his tongue against his cheek as you apply resistance.

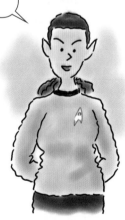

Resistance is futile. Okay, maybe not. It's actually an important part of cranial nerve assessment.

Testing the spinal accessory nerve

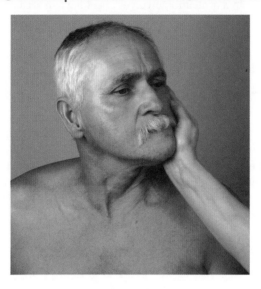

Sensory function assessment

● Sensory system evaluation involves checking five areas of sensation:

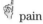 pain

 light touch

vibration

position

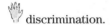 discrimination.

● Use all the major dermatomes to assess function. Each dermatome represents an area supplied with sensory fibers from an individual spinal root—cervical (C), thoracic (T), lumbar (L), or sacral (S).

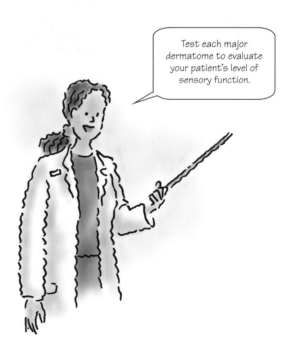

Test each major dermatome to evaluate your patient's level of sensory function.

(Text continues on page 130.)

Locating dermatomes

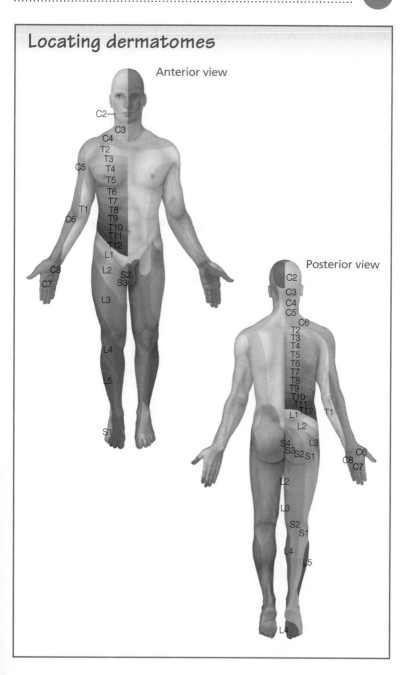

Anterior view

Posterior view

Sensory function assessment *(continued)*

Pain assessment

● Instruct the patient to close his eyes.
● Touch all the major dermatomes, first with the sharp end of a safety pin and then with the dull end.
● Follow this sequence:
  – fingers
  – shoulders
  – toes
  – thighs
  – trunk.
● If the patient has major deficits, start in the area with the least sensation and move toward the area with the most sensation to help you determine the level of deficit.

Light touch assessment

● Follow the same routine as for pain assessment, but use a wisp of cotton.

(Text continues on page 132.)

Assessing pain and light touch sensation

Pain sensation (dull stimulus)

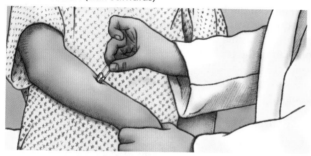

Pain sensation (sharp stimulus)

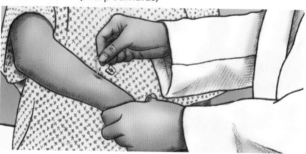

Light touch sensation

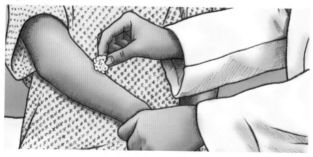

Sensory function assessment *(continued)*

Vibration assessment

- Ask the patient to close his eyes.
- Apply a vibrating tuning fork to the distal interphalangeal joint of the index finger.
- If the patient doesn't feel the sensation, moving proximally, continue to apply vibration to the joints until the patient feels the sensation.
- Repeat the test over the interphalangeal joints of the toes.

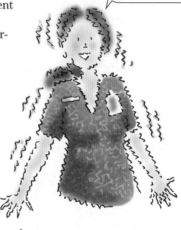

> If vibratory sense is intact, you don't have to test position sense, because the same pathway carries both senses.

Position assessment

- Ask the patient to close his eyes.
- Grasp the sides of his big toe (to test lower extremities) or index finger (to test upper extremities).
- Move the toe or finger up and down and ask the patient to identify the position.

Discrimination assessment

- Ask the patient to close his eyes.
- Place a common object—such as a coin, paper clip, or key—in the patient's hand, and ask him to identify it.
- If he can't identify the object, trace a large number on his palm and ask him to identify it.

Assessing vibration, position sense, and discrimination

Vibratory sense

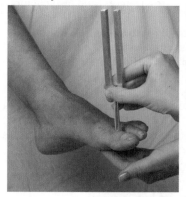

Position sense

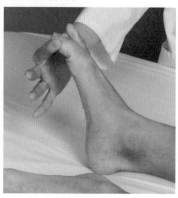

Discrimination

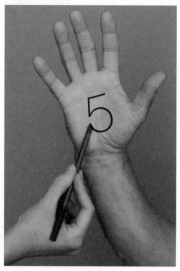

Motor function assessment

● To assess motor function, inspect the muscles and test muscle tone and strength.

● Also conduct cerebellum testing, because the cerebellum plays a role in smooth-muscle movements, such as tics, tremors, and fasciculations.

● To test arm muscle tone:
  – Move the patient's shoulder through passive range-of-motion (ROM) exercises; you should feel slight resistance.
  – Let the arm drop to the patient's side; it should fall easily.

● To test leg muscle tone:
  – Guide the hip through ROM exercises.
  – Let the leg fall to the bed; it shouldn't fall into an externally rotated position.

● Assess muscle strength by asking the patient to move major muscles against resistance.

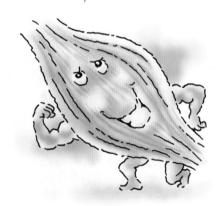

Testing muscle strength

Biceps strength

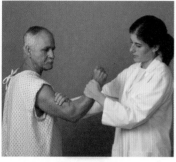

Triceps strength

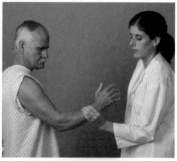

Ankle strength: Plantar flexion

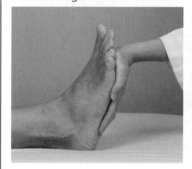

Ankle strength: Dorsiflexion

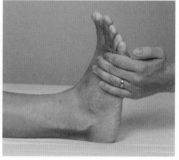

Cerebellum assessment

- Test cerebellum function:
  - Observe the patient as he walks across the room and back.
  - Ask the patient to walk heel-to-toe, and observe his balance.
  - Ask him to hop on one foot.
- Perform Romberg's test:
  - Observe the patient's balance as he stands with his eyes open, feet together, and arms at his sides.
  - Ask him to close his eyes; note his balance.
- Assess rapid alternating movements:
  - Ask the patient to touch the thumb of his right hand to his right index finger and then to each of his remaining fingers.
  - Next, ask him to sit with his palms on his thighs and ask him to turn his palms up and down, increasing in speed.

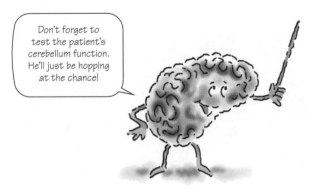

Don't forget to test the patient's cerebellum function. He'll just be hopping at the chance!

Testing balance

Tandem walking

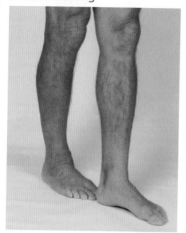

Position for Romberg's test

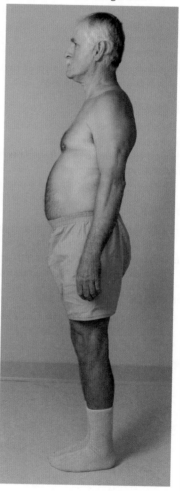

Hopping

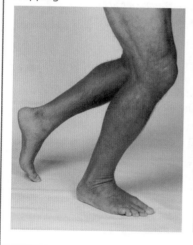

Deep tendon reflex assessment

- Test deep tendon reflexes by moving from head to toe and comparing side to side.
- Grade deep tendon reflexes using this scale:
  - 0 = Absent impulses
  - +1 = Diminished reflexes
  - +2 = Normal impulses
  - +3 = Increased impulses (may be normal)
  - +4 = Hyperactive impulses

Biceps reflex

- Position the patient's arm so that his elbow is flexed at a 45-degree angle and his arm is relaxed.
- Place your thumb over the biceps tendon and strike it with the pointed end of a reflex hammer.
- The biceps muscle should contract and the forearm should flex.

Triceps reflex

- Place the patient's forearm across his chest.
- Strike the triceps with a hammer about 2″ (5 cm) above the olecranon process on the extensor surface of the upper arm.
- The triceps muscle should contract and the forearm should extend.

Brachioradialis reflex

- Have the patient rest the ulnar surface of his hand on his abdomen or lap with his elbow partially flexed.
- Strike the radius with a hammer and watch for supination of the hand and flexion of the forearm at the elbow.

(Text continues on page 140.)

Testing biceps, triceps, and brachioradialis reflexes

Biceps reflex

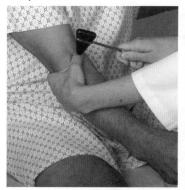

Triceps reflex

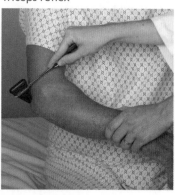

Brachioradialis reflex

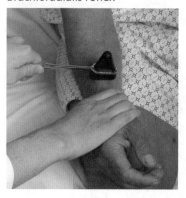

Deep tendon reflex assessment *(continued)*
Patellar reflex

- Ask the patient to sit with his legs dangling freely. If he can't sit upright, flex his knee at a 45-degree angle and place your nondominant hand behind it for support.
- Strike just below the patella with the wide end of a hammer.
- Look for contraction of the quadriceps muscle and extension of the leg.

Achilles reflex

- Ask the patient to flex his foot.
- Strike the Achilles tendon with the wide end of a hammer.
- Watch for plantar flexion of the foot at the ankle.

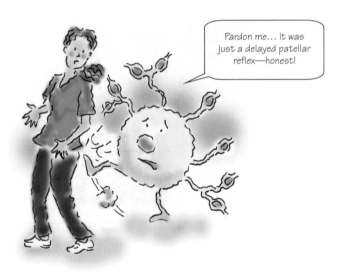

Testing patellar and Achilles reflexes

Patellar reflex

Achilles reflex

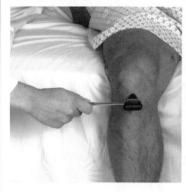
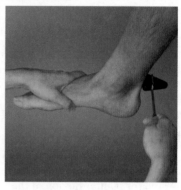

Superficial reflex assessment

● To test superficial reflexes, stimulate the skin or mucous membranes.
● Know that the more you try to elicit these cutaneous reflexes in succession, the less of a response you'll get.

Abdominal reflexes

● Have the patient lie supine with his arms at his sides and knees slightly flexed.
● Briskly stroke both sides of the abdomen above and below the umbilicus, moving from the periphery toward the midline. Look for movement of the umbilicus toward the stimulus.

Plantar response

● Using an applicator stick or tongue blade, slowly stroke the latent side of the patient's sole from the heel to the great toe.
● Watch for plantar flexion of the toes.
● Dorsiflexion or upward movement of the great toe and fanning of the little toes is an abnormal response called *Babinski's reflex*.

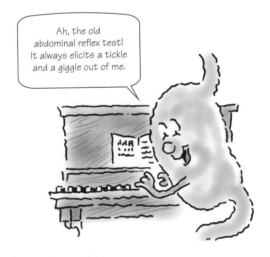

Identifying plantar response

Normal toe flexion

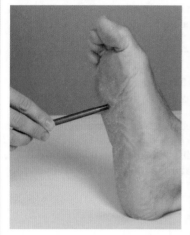

Positive Babinski's reflex

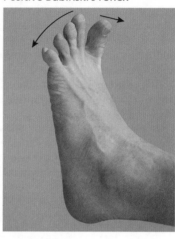

Pupillary changes

● Assess for pupillary changes to detect signs of neurologic dysfunction:

– Small pupils indicate disruption of sympathetic nerve supply to the head caused by a spinal cord lesion above T1.

– Large pupils that are bilaterally fixed and dilated indicate severe midbrain damage, hypoxia caused by cardiopulmonary arrest, or anticholinergic poisoning.

– Midposition, or slightly dilated, fixed pupils are characteristic of pressure to the midbrain caused by edema, hemorrhage, an infarction, or a contusion.

– One large pupil, fixed and dilated, is a warning sign of herniation of the temporal lobe, which can cause CN II compression. It may also indicate brain stem compression from an aneurysm, increased ICP, or head trauma with subsequent subdural or epidural hematoma.

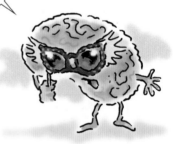

Pupillary changes can unmask conditions that cause damage to, or interfere with, CN II function.

Recognizing pupillary changes

Small pupils

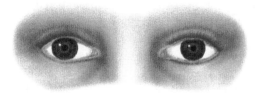

Large pupils

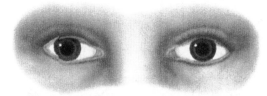

Midposition fixed pupils

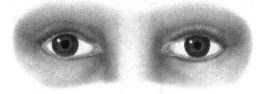

One large pupil

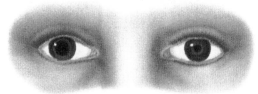

Vision impairment

● Vision defects can result from tumors or infarcts of the optic nerve head, optic chiasm, or optic tracts.

● If the patient's pupillary response to light is affected, the oculomotor nerve may be damaged.

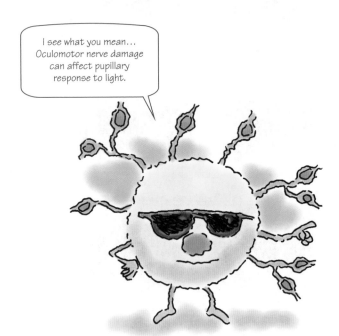

Looking at visual field deficits

	Left	Right
A: Blindness of right eye		
B: Bitemporal hemianopsia, or loss of one-half of the visual field		
C: Left homonymous hemianopsia		
D: Left homonymous hemianopsia, superior quadrant		

The black areas in these illustrations represent the field of vision loss.

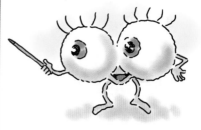

Speech impairment

- Aphasia is a speech disorder caused by injury to the cerebral cortex:
  - Expressive, or Broca's, aphasia is characterized by impaired fluency and difficulty finding words.
  - Receptive, or Wernicke's, aphasia is characterized by inability to understand written words or speech and the use of made-up words.
  - Global aphasia is characterized by a lack of expressive and receptive language.

Identifying areas of the brain affected by aphasia

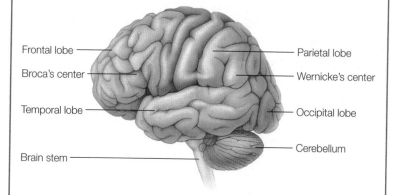

Frontal lobe

Broca's center

Temporal lobe

Brain stem

Parietal lobe

Wernicke's center

Occipital lobe

Cerebellum

Posture

Decerebrate posture

- Arms are adducted and extended, with the wrists pronated and fingers flexed.
- Legs are stiff and extended, with plantar flexion of the feet.
- This posture occurs with damage to the upper brain stem.

Decorticate posture

- Arms are adducted and flexed, with the wrists and fingers flexed on the chest.
- Legs are stiffly extended and internally rotated, with plantar flexion of the feet.
- This posture occurs with damage to one or both corticospinal tracts.

Abnormal posturing, as shown here, signals damage to the upper brain stem or one or both corticospinal tracts.

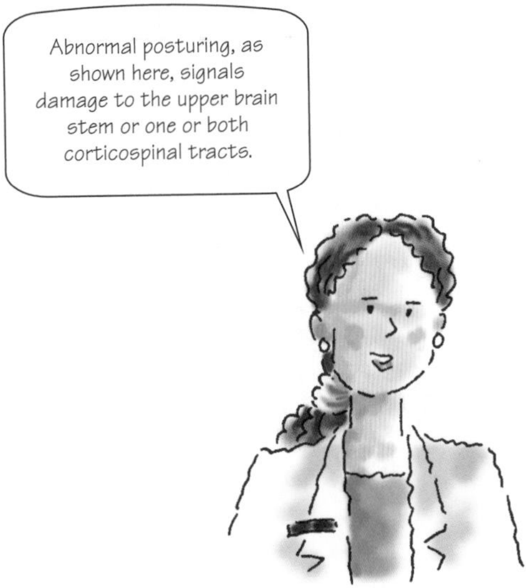

Distinguishing types of posturing

Decerebrate posture

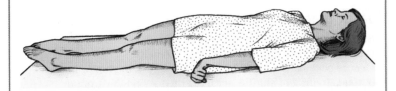

Decorticate posture

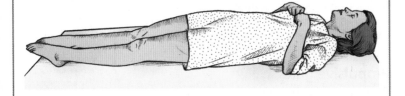

Gait abnormalities

● Gait abnormalities can result from disorders of the cerebellum, posterior columns, corticospinal tract, basal ganglia, and lower motor neurons.

Spastic gait

● Stiff, foot-dragging walk
● Caused by unilateral leg muscle hypertonicity
● Occurs because leg doesn't swing normally at the hip or knee, so the foot tends to drag or shuffle, scraping the toes on the ground

Scissors gait

● Appears as legs slightly flexing at the hips and knees, making the patient look as if he's crouching
● Causes a scissors-like movement with each step as the thighs adduct and the knees cross or hit

Propulsive gait

● Characterized by a stooped, rigid posture, with:
  – head and neck bent forward
  – flexed, stiffened arms held away from the body
  – extended fingers
  – stiffly bent knees and hips.

Steppage gait

● Typically results from footdrop
● Characterized by outward rotation of the hip and exaggerated knee flexion to lift the advancing leg off the ground
● Produces an audible slap, because the foot is thrown forward and the toes hit the ground first

Waddling gait

● Characterized by a duck-like walk

The way a patient walks can reveal important information about his neurologic status.

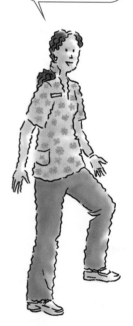

Identifying gait abnormalities

Spastic gait

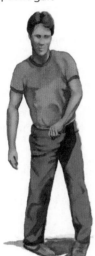

Scissors gait

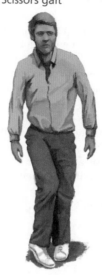

Propulsive gait

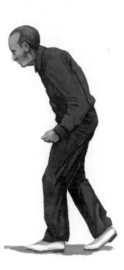

Steppage gait

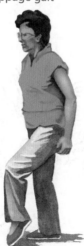

Waddling gait

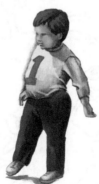

Meningeal irritation

● Positive Kernig's and Brudzinski's signs indicate meningeal irritation, which can occur with meningitis.
● To evaluate Kernig's sign:
　– Place the patient in a supine position.
　– Flex the leg at the hip and knee; then try or extend the leg while keeping the hip flexed.
　– If the patient experiences pain or spasm in the hamstring muscle and resists further extension, assume that meningeal irritation is present.
● To evaluate Brudzinski's sign:
　– Place the patient in a supine position, with your hands behind his neck.
　– Lift the patient's head toward his chest.
　– Consider the test positive if the patient flexes his ankles, knees, and hips bilaterally.
　– The patient typically complains of pain when the neck is flexed.

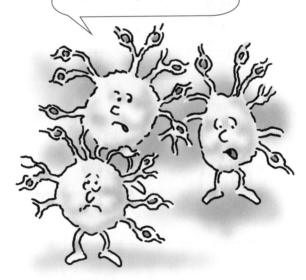

Eliciting Kernig's and Brudzinski's signs

Kernig's sign

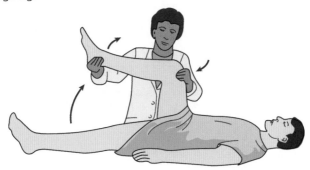

Brudzinski's sign

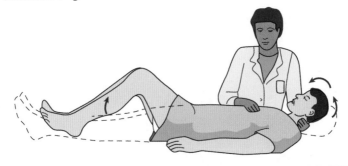

6

Respiratory system

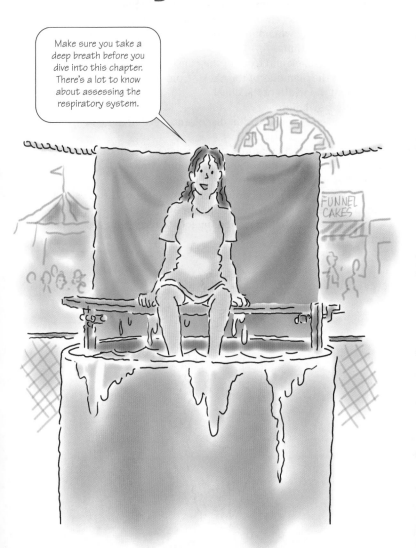

Make sure you take a deep breath before you dive into this chapter. There's a lot to know about assessing the respiratory system.

Chest inspection

- Observe the patient's breathing:
  - Count the number of breaths for a full minute. Adults normally breathe at a rate of 12 to 20 breaths/minute.
  - Note the respiratory pattern. It should be even, coordinated, and regular.
  - Observe the diaphragm and the intercostal muscles with breathing. Frequent use of accessory muscles may indicate a respiratory problem, particularly when the patient purses his lips and flares his nostrils when breathing.
- Examine the back and front of the chest:
  - Look at the diameter of the chest, from front to back. It should be about half the width of the chest
  - Look for symmetry.
  - Note masses, scars, or skin discolorations that indicate trauma or surgery.
  - Look at the costal margin (angle between the ribs and the sternum at the point immediately above the xiphoid process). The angle should be less than 90 degrees in an adult.
  - Watch for paradoxical, or uneven, movement of the chest wall, indicating loss of normal chest wall function.
- Use landmarks to help describe the locations of your assessment findings.

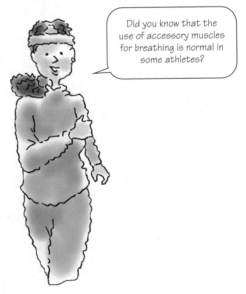

Did you know that the use of accessory muscles for breathing is normal in some athletes?

Identifying respiratory assessment landmarks

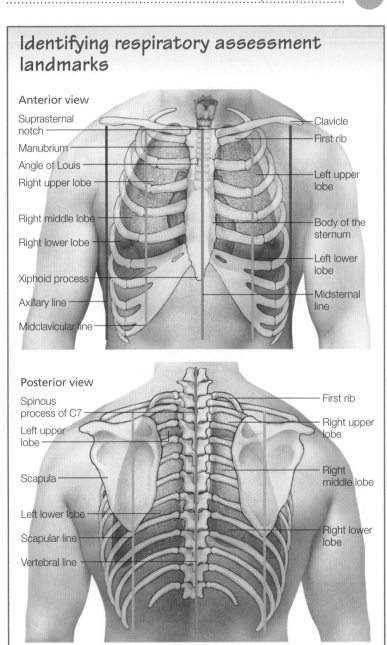

Chest palpation

● Place the palm of your hand lightly over the thorax. The chest wall should feel smooth, warm, and dry.
● Palpate for tenderness, alignment, bulging, and retractions of the chest and intercostal spaces. Gentle palpation shouldn't cause the patient pain.
● Assess the patient for crepitus, especially around drainage sites. Repeat this procedure on the patient's back.
● Use the pads of your fingers to palpate the front and back of the thorax.
● Pass your fingers over the rib cage and any scars, lumps, lesions, and ulcerations. The muscles should feel firm and smooth.
● Note the skin temperature, turgor, and moisture.

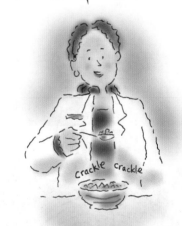

Palpating the chest

Using the palm of the hand

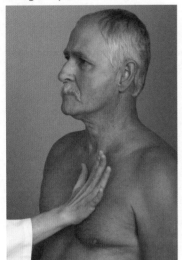

Using the pads of the fingers

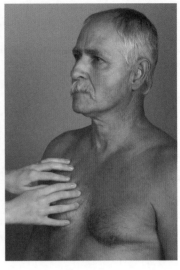

Tactile fremitus

● Ask the patient to fold his arms across his chest.
● Check for tactile fremitus by lightly placing your open palms on both sides of the patient's back, without touching his back with your fingers.
● Ask the patient to repeat the phrase "ninety-nine" loud enough to produce palpable vibrations.
● Palpate the front of the chest in the same way, using the same hand positions.

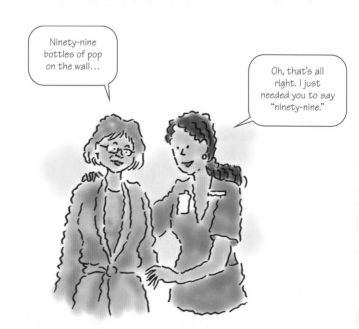

Checking for tactile fremitus

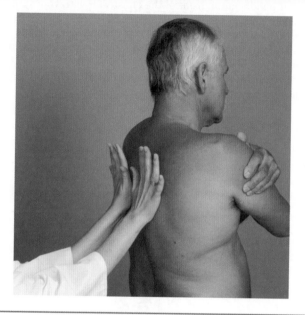

Symmetry and expansion

● Place your hands on the front of the chest wall with your thumbs touching each other at the second intercostal space.

● Instruct the patient to inhale deeply. Your thumbs should separate simultaneously and equally to a distance several centimeters away from the sternum.

● Repeat the measurement at the fifth intercostal space and on the back of the chest near the tenth rib.

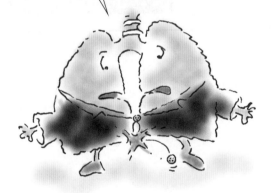

Evaluating chest wall symmetry and expansion

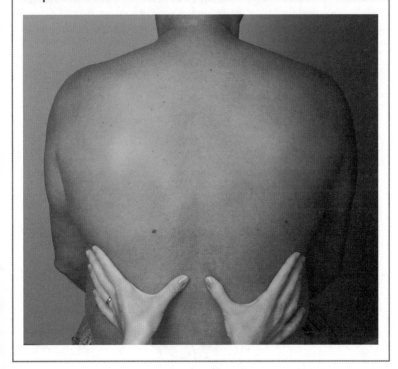

Chest percussion

- Hyperextend the middle finger of your left hand, if you're right-handed, or the middle finger of your right hand, if you're left-handed.
- Place your middle finger firmly on the patient's chest.
- Use the tip of the middle finger of your dominate hand to tap on the middle finger of your other hand just below the distal joint.

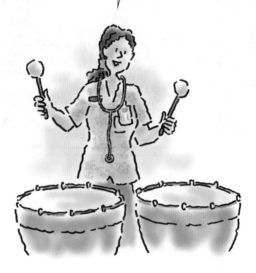

Chest percussion helps to determine the boundaries of the lungs and whether the lungs are filled with air, fluid, or solid material.

(Text continues on page 168.)

Percussing the chest

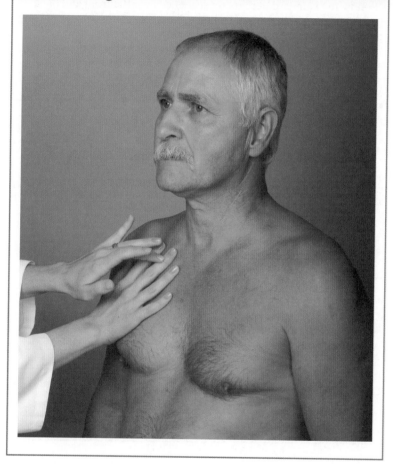

Chest percussion *(continued)*

- Follow the standard percussion sequence over the front and back chest walls. Using this sequence helps distinguish between normal and abnormal sounds in the patient's lungs.
- Compare sound vibrations from one side with those from the other, as you proceed. Different percussion sounds are heard in different areas of the chest.

Percussion sounds

Sound	Description	Clinical significance
Flat	Short, soft, high-pitched, extremely dull, found over the thigh	Consolidation, as in atelectasis and extensive pleural effusion
Dull	Medium in intensity and pitch, moderate length, thudlike, found over the liver	Solid area, as in lobar pneumonia
Resonant	Long, loud, low-pitched, hollow	Normal lung tissue; bronchitis
Hyperresonant	Very loud, lower-pitched, found over the stomach	Hyperinflated lung, as in emphysema or pneumothorax
Tympanic	Loud, high-pitched, moderate length, musical, drumlike, found over a puffed-out cheek	Air collection, as in a gastric air bubble, air in the intestines, or a large pneumothorax

Following percussion sequences

Anterior

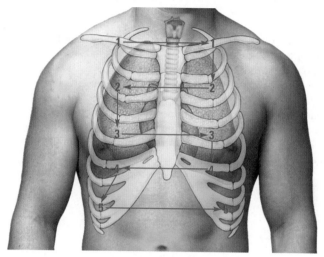

Posterior

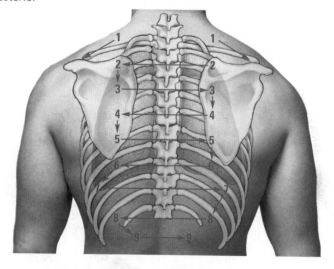

Diaphragmatic excursion

● Ask the patient to exhale.
● Percuss the back on one side to locate the upper edge of the diaphragm (the point at which normal lung resonance changes to dullness).
● Mark the spot indicating the position of the lung at full expiration on that side of the back.
● Ask the patient to inhale as deeply as possible.
● Percuss the back until you locate the diaphragm.
● Mark the spot.
● Repeat this procedure on the opposite side of the back.
● Use a ruler or tape measure to determine the distance between the marks. The distance, normally 1¼″ to 2″ (3 to 5 cm), should be equal on both the right and left sides.

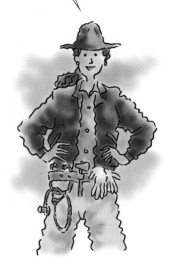

Diaphragmatic excursion is the distance the diaphragm moves between inhalation and exhalation.

Measuring diaphragm movement

Percussing the back

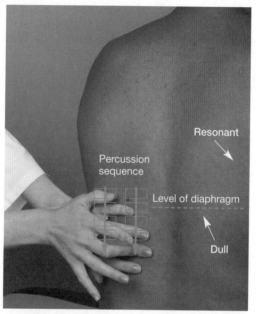

Resonant

Percussion sequence

Level of diaphragm

Dull

Measuring the distance

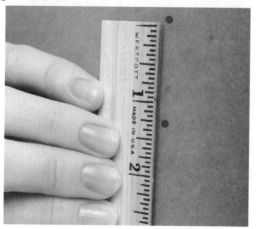

Chest auscultation

● Auscultate the lungs in the same pattern used for chest percussion (see page 169).

● Distinguish between normal and adventitious breath sounds by pressing the diaphragm of the stethoscope firmly against the skin.

● Listen to a full inspiration and a full expiration at each site in the sequence.

● Have the patient breathe through his mouth because nose breathing alters the pitch of breath sounds. The type of sound depends on where you listen.

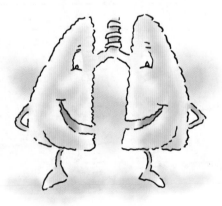

Auscultation helps you determine the condition of the alveoli and the surrounding pleurae.

Identifying locations of normal breath sounds

Anterior thorax

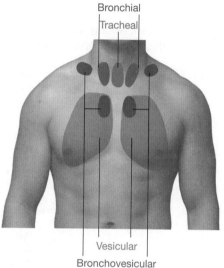

Bronchial

Tracheal

Vesicular

Bronchovesicular

Posterior thorax

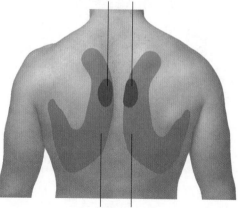

Bronchovesicular

Vesicular

Breath sounds

● Classify each sound you hear according to its intensity, location, pitch, duration, and characteristic.

● Note whether the sound occurs when the patient inhales, exhales, or both. Remember to compare sound variations from one side to the other.

● You'll hear four types of breath sounds over normal lungs:
  – vesicular—prolonged during inhalation and shortened during expiration
  – bronchial—heard loudest when the patient exhales; discontinuous
  – tracheal—heard when a patient inhales or exhales
  – bronchovesicular—heard when the patient inhales or exhales; continuous.

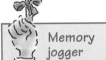

Memory jogger

To remember the qualities you'll use to classify each breath sound, think "I'll Listen Pretty Darn Closely":

Intensity

Location

Pitch

Duration

Characteristic

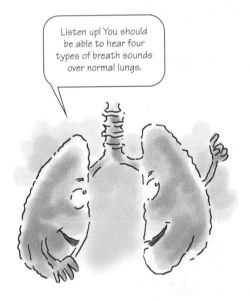

Listen up! You should be able to hear four types of breath sounds over normal lungs.

Understanding the qualities of normal breath sounds

Breath sound	Quality	Inspiration-expiration (I:E) ratio	Location
Tracheal	Harsh, high-pitched	I = E	Above supraclavicular notch, over the trachea
Bronchial	Loud, high-pitched	I < E	Just above clavicles on each side of the sternum, over the manubrium
Bronchovesicular	Medium in loudness and pitch	I = E	Next to sternum, between scapulae
Vesicular	Soft, low-pitched	I > E	Remainder of lungs

Voice sounds

- Check the patient for vocal fremitus (voice sounds resulting from chest vibrations that occur as the patient speaks). Abnormal transmissions of voice sounds may occur over consolidated areas.
- Check for bronchophony:
  - Ask the patient to say "ninety-nine" or "blue moon."
  - Over normal tissue, the words sound muffled.
  - Over consolidated areas, the words sound unusually loud and clear.
- Check for egophony:
  - Ask the patient to say the letter E.
  - Over normal tissue, the sound is muffled.
  - Over consolidated tissue, it sounds like the letter A.
- Check for whispered pectoriloquy:
  - Ask the patient to whisper "1, 2, 3."
  - Over normal tissue, the numbers are almost indistinguishable.
  - Over consolidated areas, the numbers can be heard loud and clear.

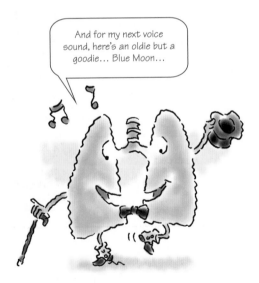

Assessing vocal fremitus

Bronchophony

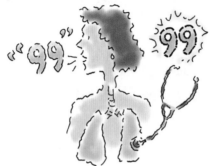

Egophony

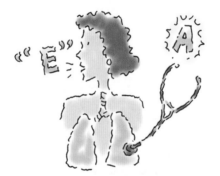

Whispered pectoriloquy

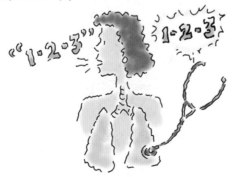

Chest wall abnormalities

Barrel chest

- Characterized by an unusually round and bulging chest, with a greater-than-normal front-to-back diameter
- Caused by chronic obstructive pulmonary disease, indicating that the lungs have lost their elasticity and that the diaphragm is flattened
- Accompanied by kyphosis of the thoracic spine, ribs that run horizontally rather than tangentially, and a prominent sternal angle

Funnel chest (pectus excavatum)

- Characterized by a funnel-shaped depression on all or part of the sternum
- May interfere with respiratory and cardiac function

If funnel chest puts the squeeze on me, you may hear a murmur during auscultation.

(Text continues on page 180.)

Looking at barrel chest and funnel chest

Barrel chest

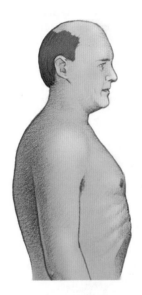

Funnel chest

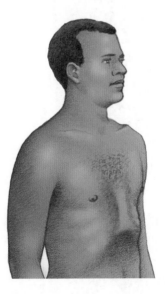

Chest wall abnormalities (continued)

Pigeon chest (pectus carinatum)

● Characterized by a displaced sternum that protrudes beyond the front of the abdomen, which increases the front-to-back diameter of the chest

Thoracic kyphoscoliosis

● Characterized by spinal curvature to one side and rotated vertebrae
● May cause difficulty assessing respiratory status because the rotation distorts the lung tissue

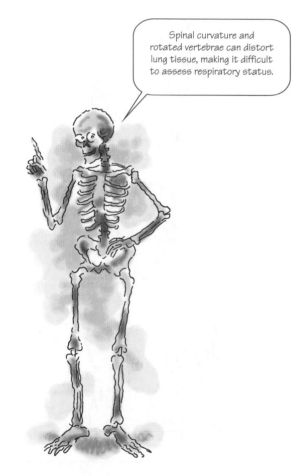

Spinal curvature and rotated vertebrae can distort lung tissue, making it difficult to assess respiratory status.

Looking at pigeon chest and thoracic kyphoscoliosis

Pigeon chest

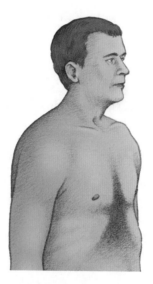

Thoracic kyphoscoliosis

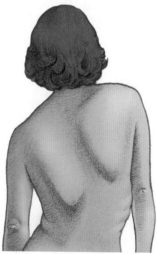

Abnormal respiratory patterns

Tachypnea

- Shallow breathing with a respiratory rate greater than 20 breaths/minute
- Commonly seen in patients with restrictive lung disease, pain, fever, sepsis, obesity, or anxiety

Bradypnea

- Decreased respiratory rate, usually below 10 breaths/minute, but regular breathing
- May be the result of central nervous system (CNS) depression caused by sedation, tissue damage, or diabetic coma

Apnea

- Absence of breathing
- May be periodic

Hyperpnea

- Deep, rapid breathing
- Can occur during or after exercise or result from pain, anxiety, or metabolic acidosis
- May indicate hypoxia or hypocalcemia in a comatose patient

(Text continues on page 184.)

Identifying tachypnea, bradypnea, apnea, and hyperpnea

Tachypnea

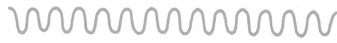

Bradypnea

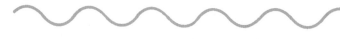

Apnea

Hyperpnea

Abnormal respiratory patterns *(continued)*

Kussmaul's respirations

- Rapid, deep, sighing breaths
- Occur in patients with metabolic acidosis, especially when it's associated with diabetic ketoacidosis
- Usually characterized by a respiratory rate greater than 20 breaths/minute and labored breath sounds

Cheyne-Stokes respirations

- Regular pattern of variations in the rate and depth of breathing in which deep breaths alternate with short periods of apnea
- Seen in patients with heart failure, kidney failure, or CNS damage

Biot's respirations

- Rapid, deep breaths that alternate with abrupt periods of apnea
- Are an ominous sign of severe CNS damage

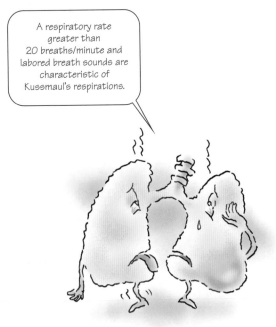

A respiratory rate greater than 20 breaths/minute and labored breath sounds are characteristic of Kussmaul's respirations.

Identifying Kussmaul's, Cheyne-Stokes, and Biot's respirations

Kussmaul's respirations

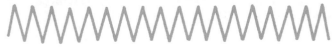

Cheyne-Stokes respirations

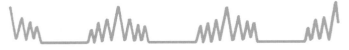

Biot's respirations

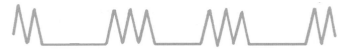

Abnormal discontinuous adventitious breath sounds

Crackles

- Caused by collapsed or fluid-filled alveoli popping open on inhalation
- Usually don't clear with coughing
- Classified as fine or coarse

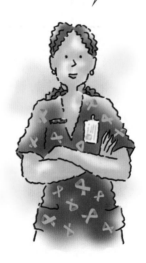

If crackles clear with coughing, they're most likely caused by secretions.

(Text continues on page 188.)

Recognizing discontinuous adventitious breath sounds

Fine crackles
- Intermittent
- Nonmusical
- Soft
- High-pitched
- Short, crackling, popping sounds
- Heard during inspiration

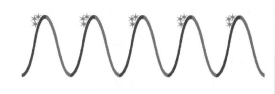

Coarse crackles
- Intermittent
- Loud
- Low-pitched
- Bubbling, gurgling sounds
- Heard during early inspiration and possibly during expiration

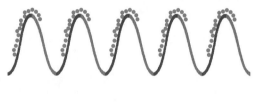

Abnormal continuous adventitious breath sounds *(continued)*

Wheezes

- High-pitched sounds heard on exhalation when airflow is blocked
- May also be heard on inspiration if the airflow blockage is severe
- Don't change with coughing

Rhonchi

- Low-pitched, snoring, or rattling sounds heard on exhalation
- May also be heard on inhalation
- Usually change or disappear with coughing, when fluid partially blocks the large airways

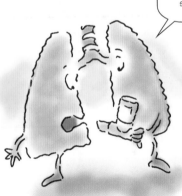

Wheezes are the unmistakably high-pitched sounds heard on exhalation when airflow is blocked, such as in someone with asthma.

Recognizing continuous adventitious breath sounds

Wheezes
- Musical
- High-pitched
- Squeaky, whistling sounds
- Heard predominantly during expiration, but may also occur during inspiration

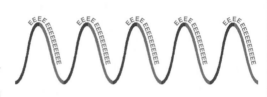

Rhonchi
- Musical
- Low-pitched
- Snoring, moaning sounds
- Heard during both inspiration and expiration, but are more predominant during expiration

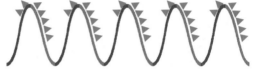

Cardiovascular system

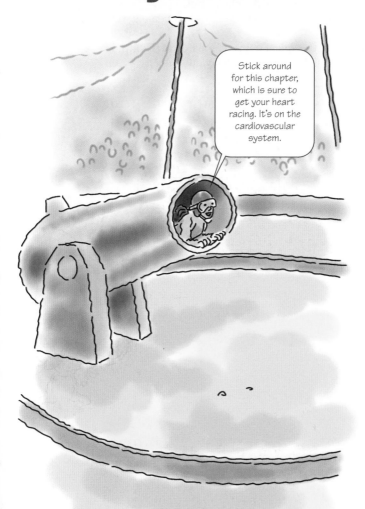

General inspection

● Take a moment to assess the patient's general appearance.
● Note the skin color, temperature, turgor, and texture. If the patient is dark-skinned, inspect the mucous membranes for pallor.
● Inspect the chest:
    – Note landmarks you can use to describe your findings as well as structures underlying the chest wall.
    – Look for pulsations, symmetry of movement, retractions, and heaves.
    – Look for the apical impulse, located at the fifth intercostal space at or just medial to the left midclavicular line.

A general inspection of the patient can provide a wealth of information about his cardiovascular status.

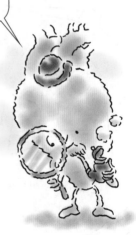

Identifying cardiovascular landmarks

Anterior thorax

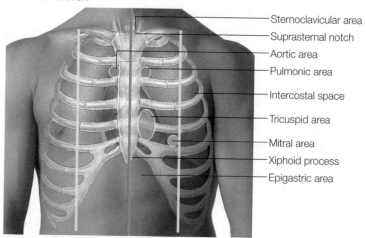

- Sternoclavicular area
- Suprasternal notch
- Aortic area
- Pulmonic area
- Intercostal space
- Tricuspid area
- Mitral area
- Xiphoid process
- Epigastric area

Lateral thorax

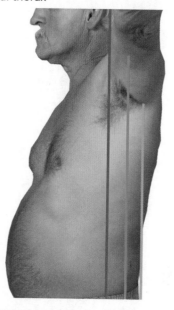

Landmark lines key
- Axillary line (anterior)
- Axillary line (posterior)
- Midaxillary line
- Midclavicular line
- Midsternal line

Heart palpation and percussion

● Palpate the apical impulse:
  – Using the ball of your hand, then your fingertips, gently palpate over the precordium to find the apical pulse.
  – Note heaves or thrills.
● If palpation is difficult with the patient lying on his back, have him lie on his side or sit upright.
● Follow a systematic palpation sequence covering the sternoclavicular, aortic, pulmonic, tricuspid, and epigastric areas. You normally won't feel pulsations in these areas.
● Percuss at the anterior axillary line and continue toward the sternum along the fifth intercostal space.
  – Sound changes from resonance to dullness over the left border of the heart, normally at the midclavicular line.
  – The right border of the heart is usually aligned with the sternum and can't be percussed.

Memory jogger

To remember the sequence for performing systematic heart palpation, think **SAP TEA**:

Sternoclavicular

Aortic

Pulmonic

Tricuspid

Epigastric

Areas.

Thrills are fine vibrations that feel like the purring of a cat.

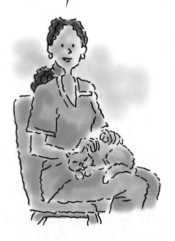

Palpating the apical impulse

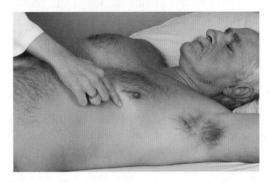

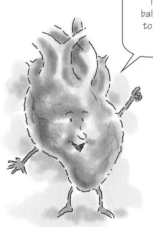

To find the apical impulse, use the ball of your hand, then your fingertips, to palpate over the precordium. Note any heaves or thrills.

Heart auscultation

● Ask the patient to breathe normally and to hold his breath periodically to enhance sounds that may be difficult to hear.
● Initially, auscultate for heart sounds with the patient in a supine position with the head of the bed raised 30 to 45 degrees.
● Begin listening at the aortic area, placing the stethoscope over the second intercostal space, along the right sternal border.
● Then move to the pulmonic area, located at the second intercostal space, at the left sternal border.
● Next, assess the tricuspid area, which lies over the fourth and fifth intercostal spaces, along the left sternal border.
● Note heart rate and rhythm, identify the first and second heart sounds (S_1 and S_2), and listen for adventitious sounds, such as third and fourth heart sounds (S_3 and S_4), murmurs, and pericardial friction rubs.
● Repeat the procedure in the opposite direction, using the bell of the stethoscope.

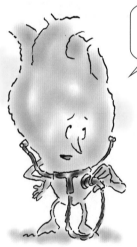

Let's see... Start with the aortic area, then move to the pulmonic area, then the tricuspid... Sounds easy enough.

Auscultating for heart sounds

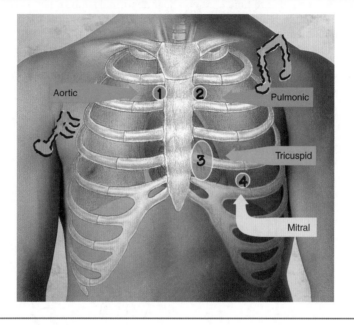

Heart auscultation positions

● If heart sounds are faint or if you hear abnormal sounds, listen again with the patient lying on his side (left lateral recumbent position) or seated and leaning forward.
● The left lateral recumbent position is best suited for hearing low-pitched sounds, using the bell of the stethoscope.
● To auscultate for high-pitched heart sounds, lean the patient forward and use the diaphragm of the stethoscope.
● To listen for pericardial friction rub:
   – Ask the patient to lean forward and exhale.
   – Listen with the diaphragm of the stethoscope over the third inter-costal space on the left side of the chest.

Use the bell of the stethoscope to hear low-pitched heart sounds and the diaphragm to hear high-pitched sounds.

Positioning the patient for auscultation

Left lateral recumbent

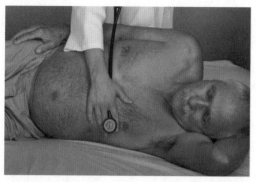

Forward leaning

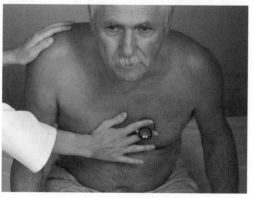

Heart sounds

- S_1:
  - Sound produced when the mitral and tricuspid valves close
  - Generally described as sounding like "lub"
  - Best heard at the base of the heart
  - Low-pitched and dull
- S_2:
  - Sound produced at the end of ventricular contraction, when the aortic and pulmonic valves snap shut
  - Generally described as sounding like "dub"
  - Shorter, higher-pitched sound than S_1
- S_3:
  - Best heard at the apex, with the patient lying on his left side
  - Commonly compared to the "y" sound in "Ken-tuck-y"
  - Commonly heard in patients with high cardiac output
  - May be a cardinal sign of heart failure in adults
- S_4:
  - Heard over the tricuspid or mitral area with the patient lying on his left side
  - Commonly described as sounding like "Ten-nes-see"
  - Occurs just before S_1, after atrial contraction
  - Indicates increased resistance to ventricular filling

Identifying heart sounds

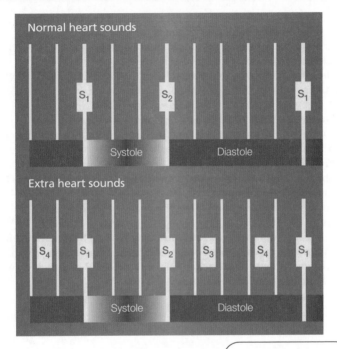

Normal heart sounds

S_1 S_2 S_1

Systole   Diastole

Extra heart sounds

S_4 S_1 S_2 S_3 S_4 S_1

Systole   Diastole

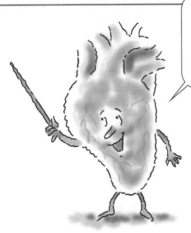

To understand where extra heart sounds fall in relation to systole, diastole, and normal heart sounds, compare these illustrations.

Vascular system inspection

- Inspect the patient's skin color.
- Note lesions, scars, and clubbing or edema of the extremities.
- Examine the fingernails and toenails for abnormalities.
- Check capillary refill; refill time should be no longer than 3 seconds.
- Evaluate the jugular vein for distension:
  - Have the patient lie on his back with the head of the bed (HOB) elevated at a 30- to 45-degree angle.
  - Ask the patient to turn his head slightly away from you.
  - Locate the angle of Louis by palpating where the clavicles join the sternum (suprasternal notch) and then sliding your fingers down the sternum until you feel a bony protuberance.
  - Find the internal jugular vein.
  - Shine a flashlight across the patient's neck to create shadows that highlight his venous pulse.
  - Locate the highest point along the vein where you can see pulsations.
  - Using a centimeter ruler, measure the distance between the high point and the sternal notch. A measurement greater than $1\frac{1}{4}''$ to $1\frac{1}{2}''$ (3 to 4 cm) above the sternal notch, with the HOB at a 45-degree angle, indicates jugular distention.

Evaluating jugular vein distention

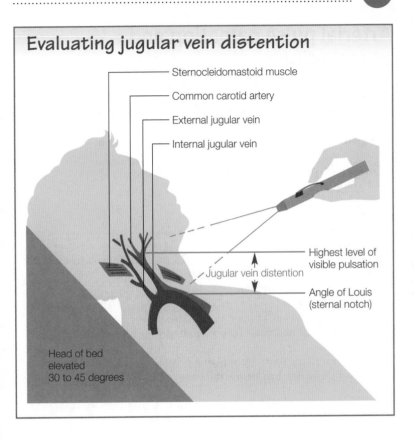

- Sternocleidomastoid muscle
- Common carotid artery
- External jugular vein
- Internal jugular vein

Highest level of visible pulsation

Jugular vein distention

Angle of Louis (sternal notch)

Head of bed elevated 30 to 45 degrees

Arterial pulse palpation and auscultation

- Start at the top of the patient's body at the temporal artery and work your way down.
- Gently press on each artery with the pads of your index and middle fingers.
- Palpate the pulse on each side, comparing pulse volume and symmetry.
- Grade each pulse on a four-point scale:
    +4 = bounding
    +3 = increased
    +2 = normal
    +1 = weak
     0 = absent.
- Palpate the carotid artery by lightly placing your fingers just medial to the trachea and below the angle of the jaw:
    - Note the rate and rhythm.
    - Assess for thrills.
    - Palpate both sides, but not at the same time.
- Palpate the brachial pulse by positioning your fingers medial to the biceps tendon.
- Palpate the radial pulse by applying pressure to the medial and ventral side of the wrist, just below the base of the thumb.

(Text continues on page 206.)

Palpating the carotid, brachial, and radial pulses

Carotid pulse

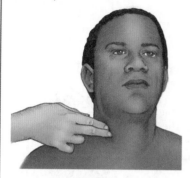

Brachial pulse

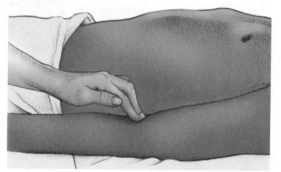

Radial pulse

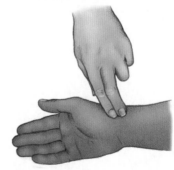

Arterial pulse palpation and auscultation *(continued)*

● To palpate the femoral pulse, press relatively hard at a point inferior to the inguinal ligament.

● To palpate the popliteal pulse, press firmly in the popliteal fossa, at the back of the knee.

● To palpate the posterior tibial pulse, apply pressure behind and slightly below the malleolus of the ankle.

● To palpate the dorsalis pedis pulse, place your fingers on the medial dorsum of the foot while the patient points his toes down. Note that the pulse is difficult to palpate here and may seem to be absent in healthy patients.

● Using the bell of the stethoscope, follow the palpation sequence and auscultate over each artery, checking for bruits and other abnormal sounds.

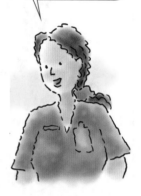

For an obese patient, you should palpate the femoral pulse in the crease of the groin, halfway between the pubic bone and hip bone.

Palpating lower extremity pulses

Femoral pulse

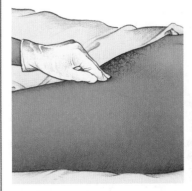

Popliteal pulse

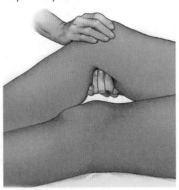

Posterior tibial pulse

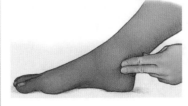

Dorsalis pedis pulse

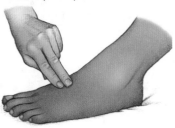

Cardiovascular abnormalities
Chest pain
- Can arise suddenly or gradually
- May initially be difficult to ascertain a cause
- Can radiate to the arms, neck, jaw, or back
- May be steady or intermittent, mild or acute
- Ranges in character from a sharp, shooting, sensation to a feeling of heaviness, fullness, or indigestion

Palpitations
- Conscious awareness of one's heartbeat described as pounding, jumping, turning, flopping, or fluttering or as missed or skipped beats
- Usually felt over the precordium or in the throat or neck
- Can be regular or irregular, fast or slow, paroxysmal or sustained

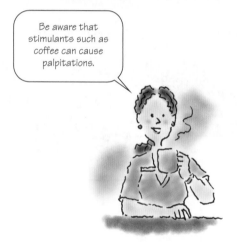

Looking at chest pain radiation sites

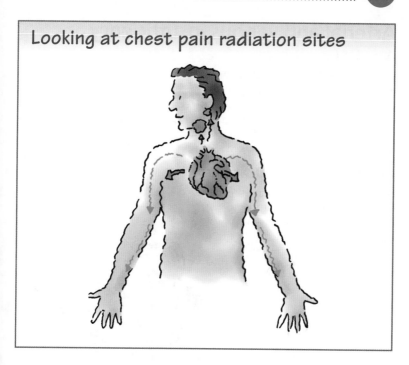

Arterial and venous insufficiency

Arterial insufficiency

- Pulses may be decreased or absent.
- Skin is cool, pale, and shiny.
- Pain may be present in the legs and feet.
- Ulcerations typically occur in the areas around the toes, and the foot usually turns deep red when dependent.
- Nails may be thick and ridged.

Chronic venous insufficiency

- Ulcerations occur around the ankle.
- Pulses are present, but may be difficult to find because of edema.
- The foot may become cyanotic when dependent.

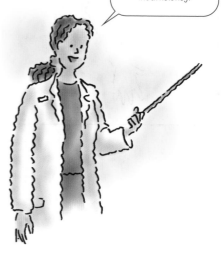

Note that your assessment findings will differ in arterial and venous insufficiency.

Recognizing arterial and venous insufficiency

Arterial insufficiency

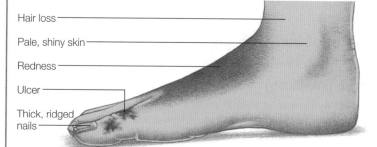

Hair loss
Pale, shiny skin
Redness
Ulcer
Thick, ridged nails

Chronic venous insufficiency

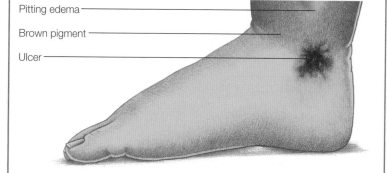

Pitting edema
Brown pigment
Ulcer

Skin and hair abnormalities

Cyanosis, pallor, and cool skin

- May indicate poor cardiac output and tissue perfusion
- Characterized by bluish or pale color in affected area and below-normal skin temperature without an associated cause, such as cold air temperature

Absence of body hair on the arms or legs

- May indicate diminished arterial blood flow to those areas

Edema (swelling)

- Caused by increased fluid in tissues
- May indicate heart failure or venous insufficiency

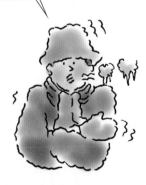

Looking at cyanosis, pallor, and edema

Cyanosis

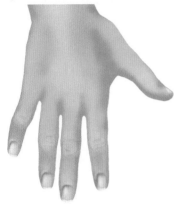

Pallor

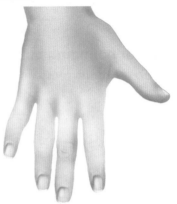

Pitting edema

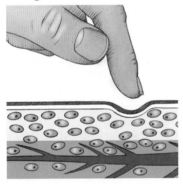

Nonpitting edema

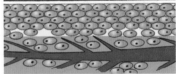
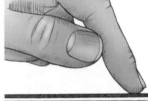

Abnormal pulsations

Weak arterial pulsations

- May indicate decreased cardiac output or increased peripheral resistance
- Points to arterial atherosclerotic disease

Strong or bounding pulsations

- Usually occur with conditions that cause increased cardiac output, such as:
    - hypertension
    - hypoxia
    - anemia
    - anxiety
    - exercise.

Thrill

- A palpable vibration
- Usually suggests valvular dysfunction

Heave

- Lifting of the chest wall felt during palpation
- Along the left sternal border, may mean right ventricular hypertrophy
- Over the left ventricular area, may mean a ventricular aneurysm

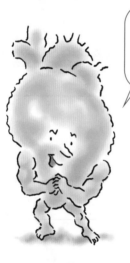

Strong or bounding pulsations aren't normal. They may signal a problem, such as hypertension, hypoxia, or anemia.

Understanding abnormal pulsations

Abnormal pulsation	What causes it
Displaced apical impulse	• Heart failure • Hypertension
Forced apical impulse	• Increased cardiac output
Aortic, pulmonic, or tricuspid pulsation	• Valvular disease • Heart chamber enlargement • Aortic aneurysm (aortic pulsation only)
Epigastric pulsation	• Heart failure • Aortic aneurysm
Sternoclavicular pulsation	• Aortic aneurysm
Slight left and right sternal pulsations	• Anemia • Anxiety • Increased cardiac output • Thin chest wall
Sternal border heave	• Right ventricular hypertrophy • Ventricular aneurysm

Abnormal pulse characteristics

Weak pulse

- Characterized by a decreased amplitude with a slow upstroke and downstroke
- May result from conditions that cause increased peripheral vascular resistance, such as heart failure, or conditions that cause decreased stroke volume, such as hypovolemia

Bounding pulse

- Characterized by a sharp upstroke, a downstroke with a pointed peak, and an elevated amplitude
- May result from conditions that increase stroke volume, such as aortic insufficiency

Pulsus alternans

- Characterized by a regular, alternating pattern of weak and strong pulses
- Associated with left-sided heart failure

Pulsus bigeminus

- Similar to pulsus alternans, but occurs at regular intervals
- Caused by premature atrial or ventricular beats

Pulsus paradoxus

- Characterized by increases and decreases in amplitude that are associated with the respiratory cycle (marked decreases occur when the patient inhales)
- Associated with pericardial tamponade and advanced heart failure

Pulsus bisferiens

- Characterized by an initial upstroke, a subsequent downstroke, and then another upstroke during systole.
- Caused by aortic stenosis and aortic insufficiency

Looking at abnormal pulse waveforms

Weak pulse

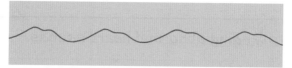

Bounding pulse

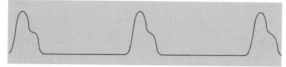

Pulsus alternans

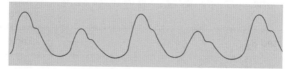

Pulsus bigeminus

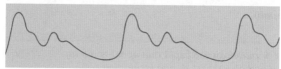

Pulsus paradoxus

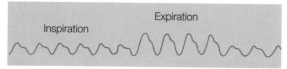

Pulsus bisferiens

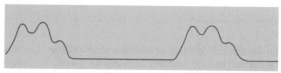

Abnormal heart sounds

- Identify sound and timing in the cardiac cycle.
- Use the characteristics to help identify possible causes.

Understanding abnormal heart sounds

Abnormal heart sound	Timing
Accentuated S_1	Beginning of systole
Diminished S_1	Beginning of systole
Split S_1 (mitral and tricuspid components to the S_1 sound)	Beginning of systole
Accentuated S_2	End of systole
Diminished or inaudible S_2	End of systole
Persistent S_2 split (aortic and pulmonic components to the S_2 sound)	End of systole
Reversed or paradoxical S_2 split that appears during exhalation and disappears during inspiration	End of systole
S_3 (ventricular gallop)	Early diastole
S_4 (atrial or presystolic gallop)	Late diastole
Pericardial friction rub (grating or leathery sound at the left sternal border; usually muffled, high-pitched, and transient)	Throughout systole and diastole

Possible causes

Mitral stenosis or fever

Mitral insufficiency, heart block, or severe mitral insufficiency with a calcified, immobile valve

Right bundle-branch block (BBB) or premature ventricular contractions

Pulmonary or systemic hypertension

Aortic or pulmonic stenosis

Delayed closure of the pulmonic valve, usually from overfilling of the right ventricle, causing prolonged systolic ejection time

Delayed ventricular stimulation, left BBB, or prolonged left ventricular ejection time

Overdistention of the ventricles during the rapid-filling segment of diastole or mitral insufficiency or ventricular failure (normal in children and young adults)

Pulmonic stenosis, hypertension, coronary artery disease, aortic stenosis, or forceful atrial contraction due to resistance to ventricular filling late in diastole (resulting from left ventricular hypertrophy)

Pericardial inflammation

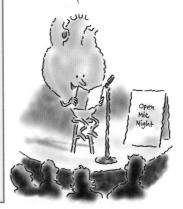

Heart murmurs

Classification

● Classify a murmur according to its timing in the cardiac cycle, its quality (blowing, musical, harsh, or rumbling), and its pitch (low, medium, or high).

● Determine where the murmur sounds loudest and grade its intensity:

1 = Barely audible

2 = Clearly audible

3 = Moderately loud

4 = Loud with palpable thrill

5 = Very loud with a palpable thrill; can be heard when the stethoscope has only partial contact with the chest

6 = Extremely loud with a palpable thrill; can be heard with the stethoscope lifted just off the chest wall.

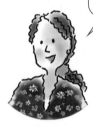

Classify your patient's murmur according to its timing, quality, and pitch and rate it on a scale of intensity from 1 to 6.

(Text continues on page 222.)

Understanding heart murmurs

Timing	Quality and pitch	Location	Possible causes
Midsystolic (systolic ejection)	Harsh, rough with medium to high pitch	Pulmonic	Pulmonic stenosis
	Harsh, rough with medium to high pitch	Aortic and suprasternal notch	Aortic stenosis
Holosystolic (pansystolic)	Harsh with high pitch	Tricuspid	Ventricular septal defect
	Blowing with high pitch	Mitral, lower left sternal border	Mitral insufficiency
	Blowing with high pitch	Tricuspid	Tricuspid insufficiency
Early diastolic	Blowing with high pitch	Midleft sternal edge (not aortic area)	Aortic insufficiency
	Blowing with high pitch	Pulmonic	Pulmonic insufficiency
Mid-diastolic to late diastolic	Rumbling with low pitch	Apex	Mitral stenosis
	Rumbling with low pitch	Tricuspid, lower right sternal border	Tricuspid stenosis

Heart murmurs *(continued)*
Murmur intensity

- Crescendo: Murmur becomes progressively louder
- Decrescendo: Murmur becomes progressively softer
- Crescendo-decrescendo: Peaks in intensity and then decreases again
- Plateau-shaped: Murmur remains equal in intensity

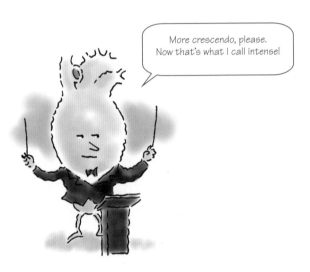

(Text continues on page 224.)

Looking at murmur configurations

Crescendo

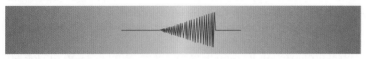

Decrescendo

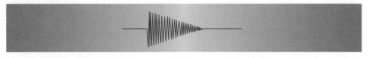

Crescendo-decrescendo

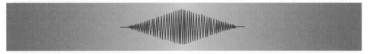

Plateau-shaped

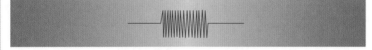

Heart murmurs *(continued)*

Common murmurs

- Aortic insufficiency: Thickened valve leaflets fail to close correctly, permitting blood backflow into the left ventricle
- Aortic stenosis: Thickened, scarred, or calcified valve leaflets impede ventricular systolic ejection
- Mitral prolapse: An incompetent mitral valve bulges into the left atrium because of an enlarged leaflet and elongated chordae tendineae
- Mitral insufficiency: Incompetent valve closure permits blood backflow into the left atrium
- Mitral stenosis: Thickened or scarred leaflets cause valve stenosis and restrict blood flow

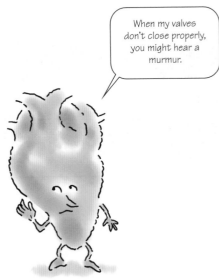

Identifying common murmurs

Aortic insufficiency (chronic)

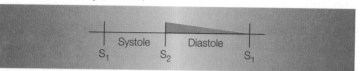

Aortic stenosis

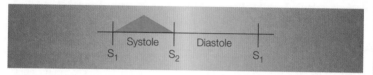

Mitral prolapse

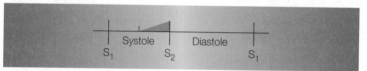

Mitral insufficiency (chronic)

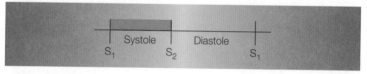

Mitral stenosis

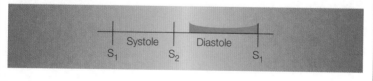

Vascular abnormalities

Venous ulcers

- Most commonly occurring leg ulcers
- Also known as *stasis ulcers*
- Result from venous hypertension
- Typically found around the ankle

Lymphatic ulcers

- Result from lymphedema, in which capillaries are compressed by thickened tissue, which occludes blood flow to the skin
- Extremely difficult to treat due to reduced blood flow

Arterial ulcers

- Result from arterial occlusive disease caused by insufficient blood flow to tissue due to arterial insufficiency
- Commonly found at the distal ends of arterial branches, especially at the tips of the toes, at the corners of nail beds, and over bony prominences

Looking at vascular ulcers

Venous ulcer

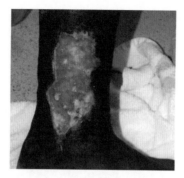

Lymphatic ulcer

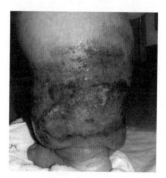

Arterial ulcer

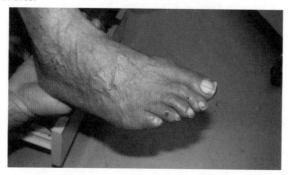

8

Gastrointestinal system

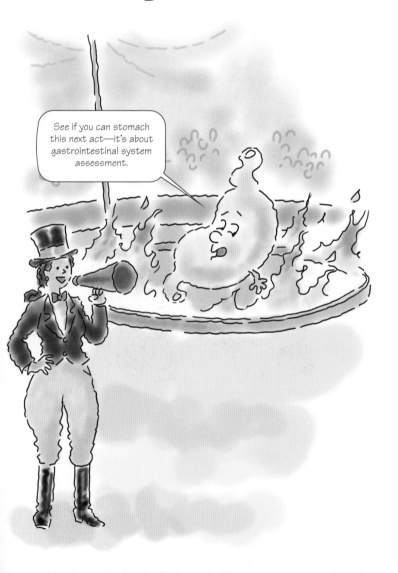

Abdominal inspection

- Mentally divide the abdomen into four quadrants, and then imagine the organs in each quadrant.
- Observe the abdomen for symmetry.
- Check for bumps, bulges, and masses.
- Observe the shape and contour. The abdomen should be flat or rounded in people of average weight and may be slightly concave in a slender person.
- Inspect the skin. It should be smooth and uniform in color.
- Record the length and appearance of any surgical scars on the abdomen.
- Note abdominal movements and pulsations.

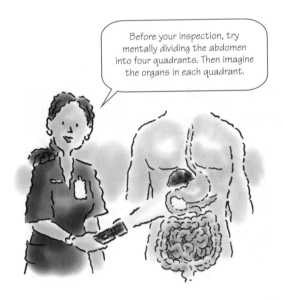

Before your inspection, try mentally dividing the abdomen into four quadrants. Then imagine the organs in each quadrant.

Identifying abdominal quadrants and structures

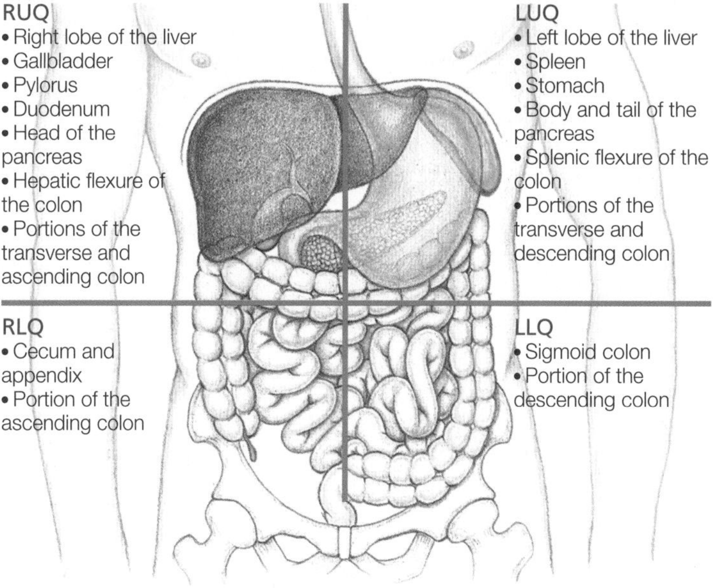

RUQ
- Right lobe of the liver
- Gallbladder
- Pylorus
- Duodenum
- Head of the pancreas
- Hepatic flexure of the colon
- Portions of the transverse and ascending colon

LUQ
- Left lobe of the liver
- Spleen
- Stomach
- Body and tail of the pancreas
- Splenic flexure of the colon
- Portions of the transverse and descending colon

RLQ
- Cecum and appendix
- Portion of the ascending colon

LLQ
- Sigmoid colon
- Portion of the descending colon

Abdominal auscultation

● Perform abdominal auscultation before percussion and palpation, because these measures can change the character of the patient's bowel sounds and lead to an inaccurate assessment.
● Auscultate in a clockwise fashion in each of the four quadrants:
  – Note the character and quality of bowel sounds in each quadrant.
  – Allow enough listening time in each quadrant before you decide that bowel sounds are absent.
  – Classify bowel sounds as normal, hypoactive, or hyperactive.
  – Normal bowel sounds are high-pitched, gurgling noises caused by air mixing with fluid during peristalsis.
● Using firm pressure, listen with the bell of the stethoscope over the aorta and the renal, iliac, and femoral arteries for bruits, venous hums, and friction rubs.

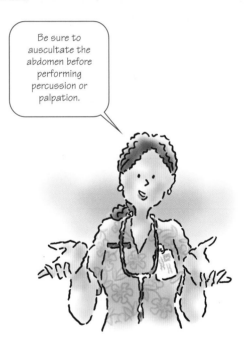

Be sure to auscultate the abdomen before performing percussion or palpation.

Identifying vascular sound locations

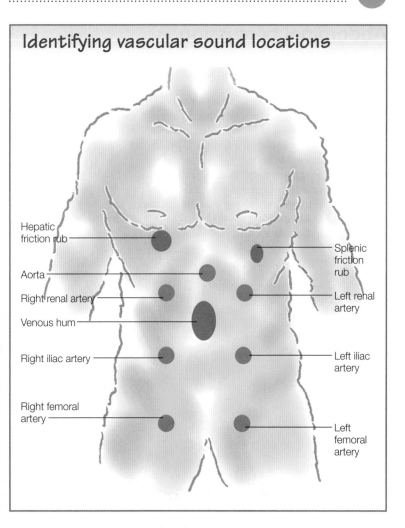

Abdominal percussion

● Use direct or indirect percussion to detect the size and location of abdominal organs and any air or fluid in the abdomen, stomach, or bowel.

● Begin percussion in the right lower abdominal quadrant and proceed clockwise, covering all four quadrants.

● Don't percuss the abdomen of a patient with an abdominal aortic aneurysm or a transplanted abdominal organ; doing so can precipitate a rupture or organ rejection.

● Two sounds are normally heard:

– **Tympany** is a clear, hollow sound that's heard over hollow organs, such as an empty stomach or bowel.

– **Dullness** is a muffled sound heard over solid organs, such as the liver, kidneys, or feces-filled intestines.

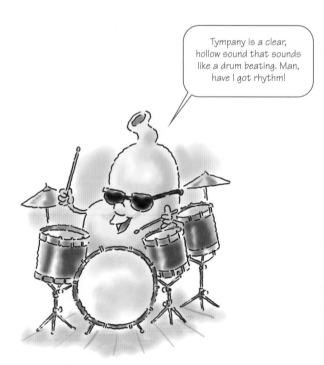

Tympany is a clear, hollow sound that sounds like a drum beating. Man, have I got rhythm!

Percussing the abdomen

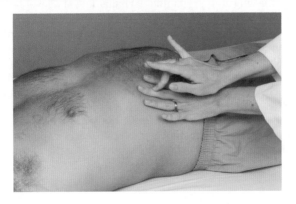

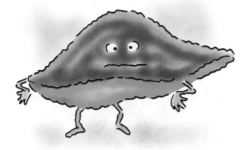

Expect to hear a muffled sound when percussing over solid organs, such as the kidneys or me. What can I say, we're a little dull.

Liver percussion and measurement

● Begin percussing at the right midclavicular line at a level below the umbilicus, and lightly percuss upward toward the liver.

● Mark the spot where the sound changes from tympany to dullness, usually at or slightly below the costal margin.

● Percuss downward along the right midclavicular line, starting above the nipple, in an area of lung resonance. Move downward until percussion notes change from normal lung resonance to dullness, usually at the fifth to seventh intercostal space.

● Use a pen to mark this spot (the upper border of the liver).

● Measure the vertical span between the two marked spots with a ruler. In an adult, a normal liver span is 4 to 8 cm at the midsternal line and 6 to 12 cm at the right midclavicular line.

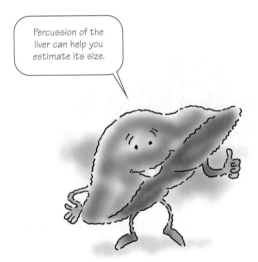

Percussion of the liver can help you estimate its size.

Measuring the liver

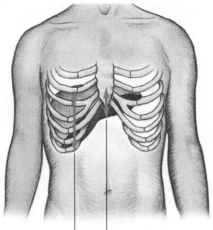

6 to 12 cm at the
right midclavicular line

4 to 8 cm at the
midsternal line

Spleen percussion

- Begin percussion at the lowest intercostal space along the left anterior axillary line; percussion notes should be tympanic.
- Ask the patient to take a deep breath, and then percuss this area again:
    - If the spleen is normal in size, the area will remain tympanic.
    - If the percussion notes change on inspiration from tympanic to dull, the spleen is probably enlarged.
- To estimate spleen size, outline the spleen's edge by percussing in several directions from areas of tympany to areas of dullness.
- Note that the spleen is difficult to percuss because tympany from the colon masks the dullness of the spleen.

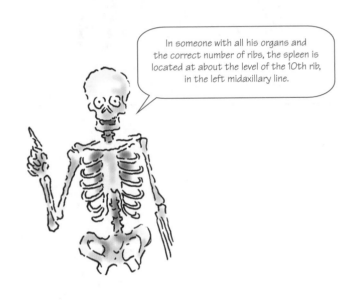

In someone with all his organs and the correct number of ribs, the spleen is located at about the level of the 10th rib, in the left midaxillary line.

Percussing the spleen

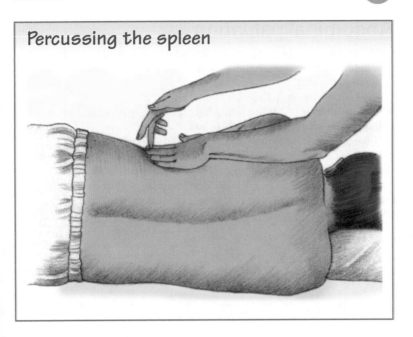

Abdominal palpation

- Abdominal palpation includes light and deep touch that helps:
  - determine the size, shape, position, and tenderness of major abdominal organs;
  - detect masses and fluid accumulation.
- Palpate all four quadrants using light and deep palpation.
- Palpate painful and tender areas last.
- Note organs, masses, and areas of tenderness or resistance.
- If the patient complains of abdominal tenderness before you touch him, palpate by lightly placing your stethoscope on his abdomen.
- If the patient's abdomen is rigid, don't palpate it. Peritoneal inflammation may be present, and palpation could cause pain or could rupture an inflamed organ.

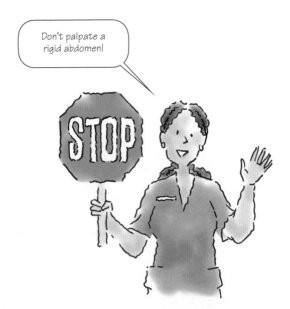

Palpating the abdomen

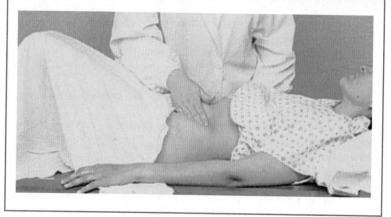

Liver palpation

Standard palpation

- Place the patient in a supine position.
- Standing on the patient's right side, place your left hand under his back at the approximate location of the liver.
- Place your right hand slightly below the mark at the liver's upper border that you made during percussion.
- Point the fingers of your right hand toward the patient's head just under the costal margin.
- As the patient inhales deeply, gently press in and up on the abdomen until the liver brushes under your right hand. The edge should be smooth, firm, and somewhat round.
- Note any tenderness.

Hooking the liver

- Stand next to the patient's right shoulder, facing his feet.
- Place your hands side by side, and hook your fingertips over the right costal margin, below the lower mark of dullness.
- Ask the patient to take a deep breath as you push your fingertips in and up. If the liver is palpable, you may feel its edge as it slides down in the abdomen as the patient inhales.

Palpating the liver

Standard palpation

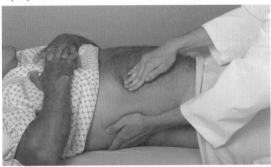

Hooking the liver

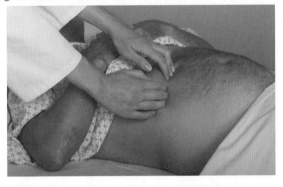

Spleen palpation

- With the patient in a supine position and you at his right side, reach across him to support the posterior lower left rib cage with your left hand.
- Place your right hand below the left costal margin and press inward.
- Instruct the patient to take a deep breath.
- Normally, the spleen isn't palpable and doesn't descend on deep inspiration below the 10th intercostal space at the posterior maxillary line.
- If the spleen is enlarged, you'll feel its rigid border. If you do feel the spleen, stop palpating immediately, because an enlarged spleen can easily rupture.

Palpating the spleen

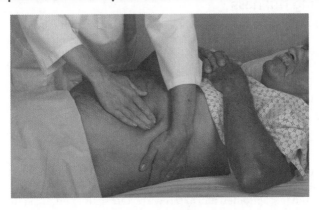

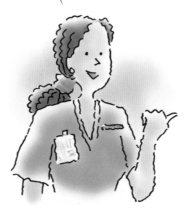

Remember to palpate for the spleen carefully, because an enlarged spleen can easily rupture.

Ascites

Shifting dullness

● With the patient in a supine position, percuss from the umbilicus outward to the flank. Draw a line on the patient's skin to mark the change from tympany to dullness.
● Turn the patient onto his side. (Note that this position causes fluid to shift). Percuss again and mark the change from tympany to dullness. Any difference between these lines might indicate ascites.

Fluid wave

● Have an assistant place the ulnar edge of her hand firmly on the patient's abdomen at its midline.
● As you stand facing the patient's head, place the palm of your left hand against the patient's right flank.
● Give the left abdomen a firm tap with your right hand. If ascites is present, you may see and feel a "fluid wave" ripple across the abdomen.
● If you detect ascites, use a tape measure to measure the fullest part of the abdomen. Mark this point on the patient's abdomen with a felt-tip marker so you'll be sure to measure it consistently. This measurement is important, especially if fluid removal or paracentesis is performed.

Testing for a fluid wave

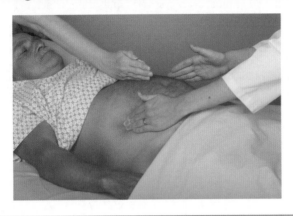

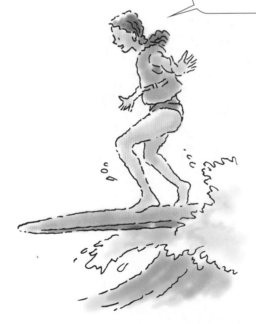

In assessment, a fluid wave isn't such a good thing. It's a sign of ascites.

Abdominal aorta assessment

● Inspect the abdominal aorta for aortic pulsation, which may indicate an aortic aneurysm.

● If no pulsatile mass is visible, palpate the upper abdomen to the left of the midline. Normally, the aortic pulsation is regular and moderately strong.

● In patients older than age 50, assess the width of the aorta by pressing firmly into the upper abdomen with one hand on each side of the aorta. The width of the aorta should be less than $1\frac{1}{4}''$ (3 cm).

Identifying the aorta

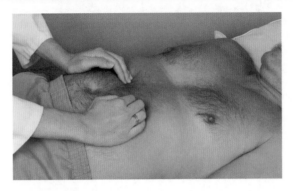

Abdominal pain assessment

Iliopsoas sign

- Help the patient into a supine position with his legs straight.
- Instruct him to raise his right leg upward as you exert slight downward pressure with your left hand on his right thigh.
- Repeat this maneuver with the left leg.
- Presence of abdominal pain, a positive result, indicates irritation of the psoas muscle and possibly appendicitis or peritonitis.

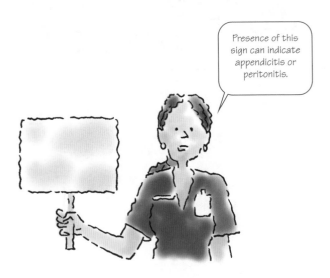

Presence of this sign can indicate appendicitis or peritonitis.

(Text continues on page 252.)

Eliciting the iliopsoas sign

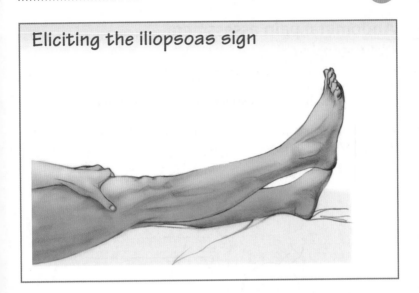

Abdominal pain assessment *(continued)*
Obturator sign

● Help the patient into a supine position with his right leg flexed 90 degrees at the hip and knee.
● Hold the leg above the knee and at the ankle; then rotate the leg laterally and medially.
● Pain in the hypogastric region is a positive sign, indicating irritation of the obturator muscle.

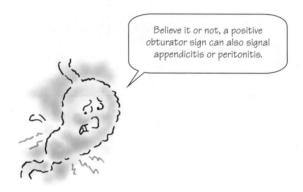

Believe it or not, a positive obturator sign can also signal appendicitis or peritonitis.

(Text continues on page 254.)

Eliciting the obturator sign

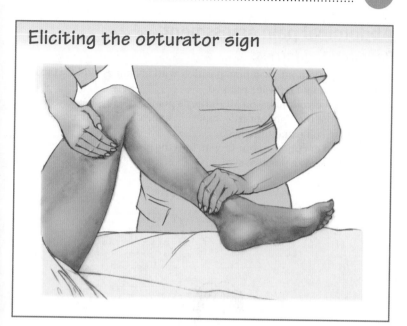

Abdominal pain assessment *(continued)*
Rebound tenderness

● Help the patient into a supine position with his knees slightly flexed and his abdominal muscles relaxed.
● Gently place your hand on McBurney's point, which is located about 2″ (5 cm) from the right anterior superior spine of the ilium, on a line between the spine and umbilicus.
● Slowly and deeply dip your fingers into the area and then release. Pain on release is a positive sign.

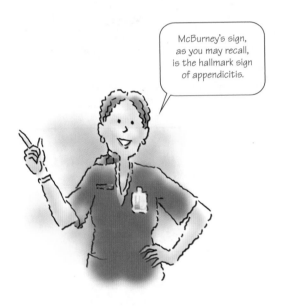

McBurney's sign, as you may recall, is the hallmark sign of appendicitis.

Eliciting rebound tenderness

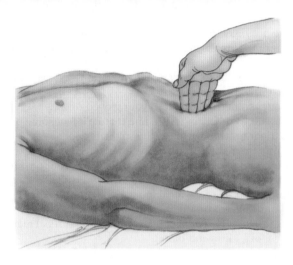

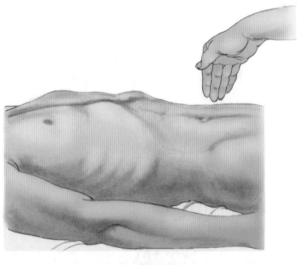

Rectum and anus examination

- If your patient is age 40 or older, perform a rectal examination.
- Put on gloves.
- Spread the buttocks to expose the anus and surrounding tissue. The skin in the perineal area is normally somewhat darker than that of the surrounding area.
- Check for fissures, lesions, scars, inflammation, discharge, rectal prolapse, and external hemorrhoids.
- Apply a water-soluble lubricant to your gloved finger.
- Tell the patient to relax, and warn him that he'll feel some pressure.
- Ask the patient to bear down. As the sphincter opens, gently insert your finger into the rectum, toward the umbilicus.
- To palpate as much of the rectal wall as possible, rotate your finger clockwise and then counterclockwise. The rectal wall should feel soft and smooth, without masses, fecal impaction, or tenderness.
- Remove your finger from the rectum.
- Inspect the glove for stool, blood, and mucus. Test fecal matter adhering to the glove for occult blood.

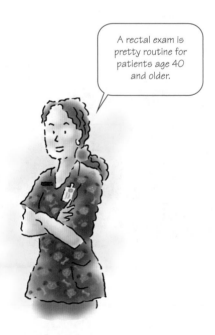

A rectal exam is pretty routine for patients age 40 and older.

Examining the rectum and anus

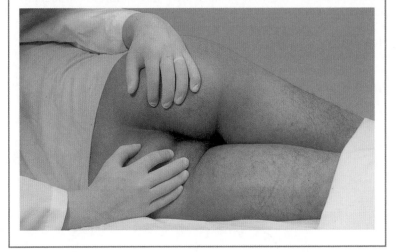

Abdominal distention

- Results from increased abdominal pressure that forces the abdominal wall outward
- May be caused by gas, a tumor, a colon filled with feces, or an incisional hernia
- Can be mild or severe, depending on the amount of pressure
- Can be localized or diffuse
- Can occur suddenly or gradually

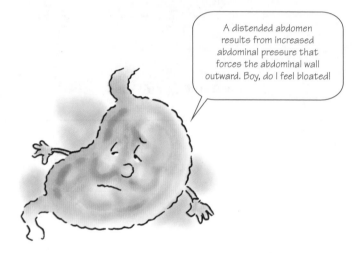

A distended abdomen results from increased abdominal pressure that forces the abdominal wall outward. Boy, do I feel bloated!

Looking at abdominal distention

Gas

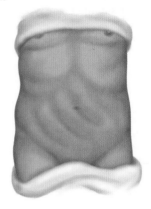

Tumor

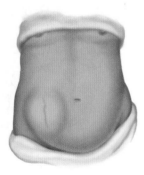

Incisional hernia

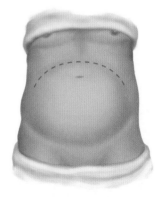

Abdominal pain

- May indicate ulcers, intestinal obstruction, appendicitis, cholecystitis, peritonitis, or another inflammatory disorder
- May be described as burning, cramping, or stabbing (the type of pain is a clue to its cause)
- May radiate to other areas

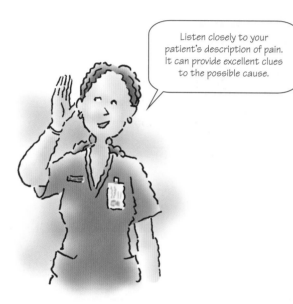

Listen closely to your patient's description of pain. It can provide excellent clues to the possible cause.

Identifying causes of abdominal pain

Type of abdominal pain	Possible cause
Burning	• Peptic ulcer • Gastroesophageal reflux disease
Cramping	• Biliary colic • Irritable bowel syndrome • Diarrhea • Constipation • Flatulence
Severe cramping	• Appendicitis • Crohn's disease • Diverticulitis
Stabbing	• Pancreatitis • Cholecystitis

Identifying abdominal pain origins

Affected organ	Visceral pain
Stomach	Midepigastrium
Small intestine	Periumbilical area
Appendix	Periumbilical area
Proximal colon	Periumbilical area and right flank for ascending colon
Distal colon	Hypogastrium and left flank for descending colon
Gallbladder	Midepigastrium
Ureters	Costovertebral angle
Pancreas	Midepigastrium and left upper quadrant
Ovaries, fallopian tubes, and uterus	Hypogastrium and groin

After you assess the location of a patient's pain, use this chart to get an idea of the most likely source of the pain.

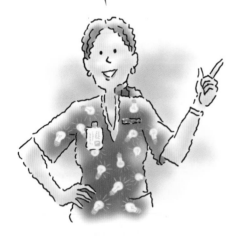

Parietal pain	Referred pain
Midepigastrium and left upper quadrant	Shoulders
Over affected site	Midback (rare)
Right lower quadrant	Right lower quadrant
Over affected site	Right lower quadrant and back (rare)
Over affected site	Left lower quadrant and back (rare)
Right upper quadrant	Right subscapular area
Over affected site	Groin; scrotum in men, labia in women (rare)
Midepigastrium and left upper quadrant	Back and left shoulder
Over affected site	Inner thighs

Abnormal abdominal sounds

Hyperactive bowel sounds

- Commonly characterized as rapid, rushing, gurgling waves of sound
- Sometimes audible without a stethoscope
- Reflect increased intestinal motility

Hypoactive bowel sounds

- Are less regular, frequent, and loud than normal bowel sounds
- Occur normally during sleep
- Reflect decreased intestinal motility

Absent bowel sounds

- Inability to hear any bowel sounds with a stethoscope for at least 5 minutes in every quadrant
- May be caused by mechanical or vascular obstruction or neurogenic inhibition that halts peristalsis

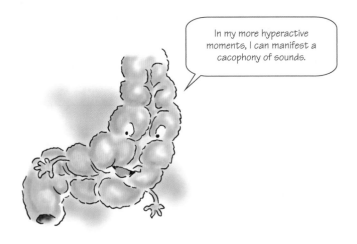

Identifying abnormal abdominal sounds

Sound and description	Location	Possible cause
Abnormal bowel sounds		
Hyperactive sounds (unrelated to hunger)	Any quadrant	Diarrhea, laxative use, or early intestinal obstruction
Hypoactive, then absent sounds	Any quadrant	Paralytic ileus or peritonitis
High-pitched tinkling sounds	Any quadrant	Intestinal fluid and air under tension in a dilated bowel
High-pitched rushing sounds coinciding with abdominal cramps	Any quadrant	Intestinal obstruction (life-threatening)
Systolic bruits		
Vascular blowing sounds resembling cardiac murmurs	Over abdominal aorta	Partial arterial obstruction or turbulent blood flow
	Over renal artery	Renal artery stenosis
	Over iliac artery	Iliac artery stenosis
Venous hum		
Continuous, medium-pitched tone created by blood flow in a large engorged vascular organ such as the liver	Epigastric and umbilical regions	Increased collateral circulation between portal and systemic venous systems, such as in cirrhosis
Friction rub		
Harsh, grating sound like two pieces of sandpaper rubbing together	Over liver and spleen	Inflammation of the peritoneal surface of the liver, such as from a tumor

9

Genitourinary system

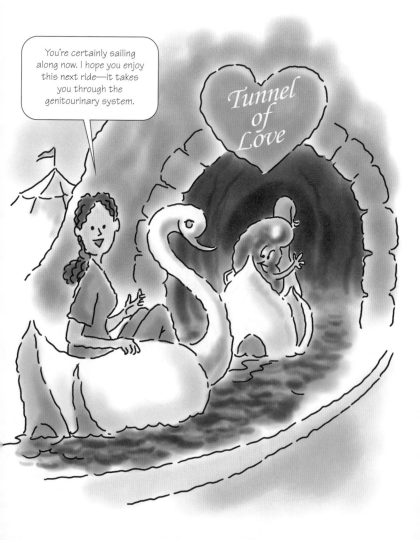

Kidney palpation

● Ask the patient to lie in a supine position.
● Standing on the patient's right side, place your left hand under the patient's back and your right hand on his abdomen.
● Instruct the patient to inhale deeply, so the kidney moves downward.
● Pull up with your left hand and press down with your right hand as the patient inhales.
● Reach across the patient's abdomen, placing your left hand behind the left flank to palpate the left kidney.
● Place your right hand over the area of the left kidney.
● Ask the patient to inhale deeply again.
● Pull up with your left hand and press down with your right as the patient inhales.

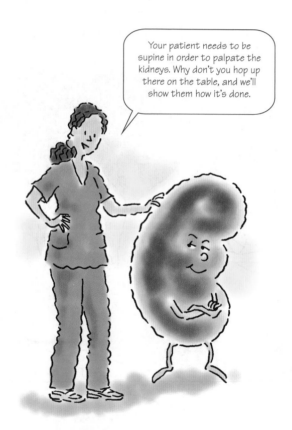

Palpating the kidneys

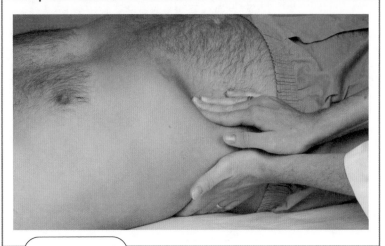

Keep in mind that you can't usually palpate the kidneys unless they're enlarged.

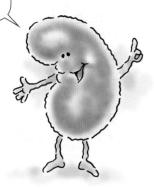

Kidney percussion

- Ask the patient to sit upright.
- Place the ball of your nondominant hand on the patient's back at the costovertebral angle of the 12th rib.
- Strike the ball of your nondominant hand with the ulnar surface of your dominant hand. Use just enough force to cause a painless but perceptible thud.

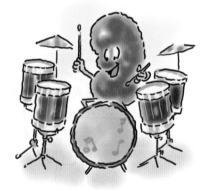

Kidney percussion can be used to check for costovertebral angle tenderness, a sign of inflammation.

Percussing the kidneys

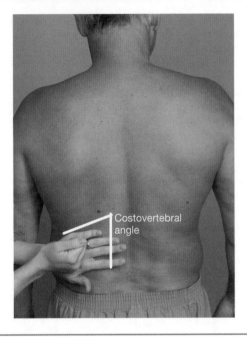

Costovertebral angle

External female genitalia inspection

- Put on a pair of gloves.
- Inspect the external genitalia and pubic hair to assess sexual maturity.
- Spread the labia and locate the urethral meatus. Note the presence of discharge or ulcerations.
- Using your index finger and thumb, gently spread the labia majora and minora.
    - The area should be moist and free from lesions.
    - You may detect a normal discharge that varies from clear and stretchy before ovulation to white and opaque after ovulation; it should be odorless and nonirritating to the mucosa.
- Examine the vestibule, especially the area around the Bartholin's and Skene's glands.
    - Check for swelling, redness, lesions, discharge, and unusual odor.
    - If any of these unusual conditions exist, obtain a specimen for culture.
- Inspect the vaginal opening, noting whether the hymen is intact or perforated.

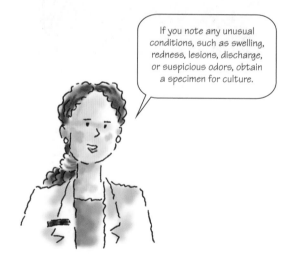

If you note any unusual conditions, such as swelling, redness, lesions, discharge, or suspicious odors, obtain a specimen for culture.

Inspecting the genitalia

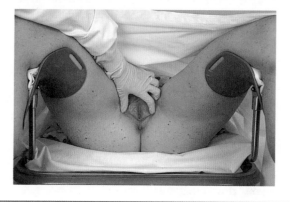

External female genitalia palpation

- Spread the labia with one hand and palpate with the other.
  - The labia should feel soft, and the patient shouldn't feel any pain.
  - Note swelling, hardness, or tenderness.
  - If you detect a mass or lesion, palpate it to determine the size, shape, and consistency.
- If you find swelling or tenderness, see if you can palpate the Bartholin's glands, which normally aren't palpable:
  - Carefully insert your finger into the patient's posterior introitus.
  - Place your thumb along the lateral edge of the swollen or tender labium.
  - Gently squeeze the labium.
  - If discharge from the duct results, culture it.
- If the urethra is inflamed, milk it and the area of the Skene's glands:
  - Moisten your gloved finger with water.
  - Separate the labia with your other hand.
  - Insert your index finger about 1¼″ (3 cm) into the anterior vagina.
  - Continue palpating down to the introitus, keeping in mind that this procedure shouldn't cause the patient discomfort.
  - Culture any discharge.

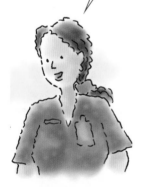

Be sure to warn the patient before you touch her. It may help her to feel more comfortable with the examination.

Palpating Bartholin's glands

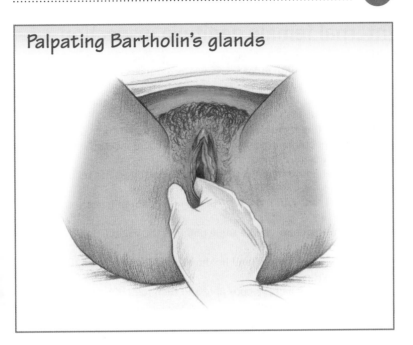

Internal female genitalia inspection

- Select an appropriate speculum for your patient's size and shape.
- Rinse the speculum under warm water to lubricate and warm the blades.
- With gloved hands, place the index and middle fingers of your dominant hand about 1″ (2.5 cm) into the vagina.
- Spread the fingers to exert pressure on the posterior vagina.
- Hold the speculum in your dominant hand, and insert the blades between your fingers.
- Ask the patient to bear down to open the introitus and relax the perineal muscles.
- Insert the blades until the base of the speculum touches your fingers, inside the vagina.
- Rotate the speculum in the same plane as the vagina, and withdraw your fingers.
- Using the thumb of the hand holding the speculum, press the lower lever to open the blades.
- Open the blades as far as possible and then lock them by tightening the thumb screw above the lever.

Inserting a speculum

Initial insertion

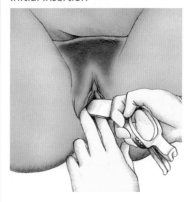

Deeper insertion

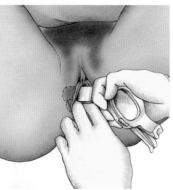

Rotation and opening

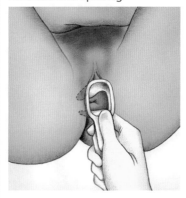

Vaginal and cervical inspection

- Observe the color, texture, and integrity of the vaginal lining.
  - A thin, white, odorless discharge on the vaginal walls is normal.
- Examine the cervix for color, position, size, shape, mucosal integrity, and discharge.
  - The cervix should be smooth and round.
- Inspect the central cervical opening, or cervical os.
  - The os is circular in a woman who hasn't given birth vaginally (nulliparous) and is a horizontal slit in a woman who has (parous).
  - Expect to see a clear, watery cervical discharge during ovulation and a slightly bloody discharge just before menstruation.
- Obtain a specimen for a Pap test.
- Unlock and close the blades of the speculum, and then withdraw the speculum.

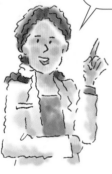

Expect the cervical os to appear circular in a woman who hasn't given birth vaginally and as a horizontal slit in a woman who has.

Looking at the cervical os

Nulliparous

Parous

Internal genitalia palpation

● Lubricate the index and middle fingers of your gloved dominant hand.

● Use the thumb and index finger of your other hand to spread the labia majora.

● Insert your two lubricated fingers into the vagina, exerting pressure posteriorly to avoid irritating the anterior wall and urethra.

● Note tenderness or nodularity in the vaginal wall.

● Sweep your fingers from side to side across the cervix and around the os.

– The cervix should move in all directions.

Palpating the vagina and cervix

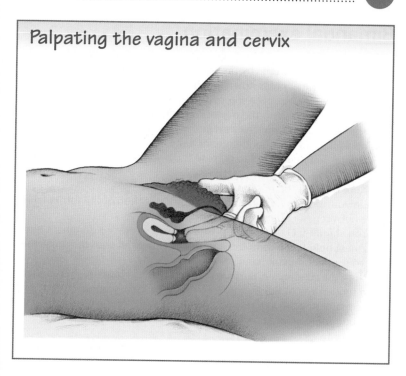

Bimanual examination

● With the index and middle fingers of your gloved dominant hand, elevate the cervix and uterus by pressing upward inside the vagina.

● At the same time, press down and in with your hand on the abdomen; try to grasp the uterus between your hands.

● Move your fingers into the posterior fornix (the recessed space behind the cervix), pressing upward and forward to bring the anterior uterine wall up to your nondominant hand.

● Use your dominant hand to palpate the lower portion of the uterine wall.

    – Note the position of the uterus.

● Slide your fingers further into the anterior section of the fornix (the space between the uterus and the cervix).

    – You should feel part of the posterior wall with your dominant hand.

    – You should feel part of the anterior uterine wall with the fingertips of your nondominant hand.

    – Note the size, shape, surface characteristics, consistency, motility, and tenderness of the uterus.

● After palpating the anterior and posterior walls of the uterus, move your nondominant hand toward the right lower quadrant of the abdomen.

● Slip the fingers of your dominant hand into the right fornix and palpate the right ovary; then palpate the left ovary.

    – Note the size, shape, and contour of each ovary.

    – Know that the ovaries might not be palpable in women who aren't relaxed or are obese.

    – Also keep in mind that the ovaries shouldn't be palpable in postmenopausal women.

● Remove your hand from the patient's abdomen and your fingers from her vagina.

● Discard your gloves, unless you're also performing a rectovaginal examination.

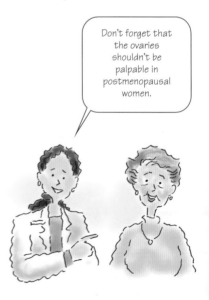

Don't forget that the ovaries shouldn't be palpable in postmenopausal women.

Performing a bimanual exam

Palpating the uterus

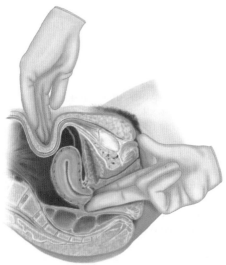

Palpating the ovaries

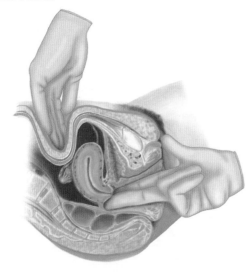

Rectovaginal examination

● Apply water-soluble lubricant to your gloved index and middle fingers of your dominant hand.
● Instruct the patient to bear down with her vaginal and rectal muscles.
● Insert your index finger a short way into the vagina and your middle finger into the rectum.
● Use your middle finger to assess rectal muscle and sphincter tone.
● Insert your middle finger deeper into the rectum and palpate the rectal wall.
● Sweep the rectum with your finger, assessing for masses or nodules.
● Palpate the posterior wall of the uterus through the anterior wall of the rectum, evaluating the uterus for size, shape, tenderness, and masses.
  – The rectovaginal septum (wall between the rectum and vagina) should feel smooth and springy.
● Place your nondominant hand on the patient's abdomen at the symphysis pubis.
● With your index finger in the vagina, palpate deeply to feel the posterior edge of the cervix and the lower posterior wall of the uterus.
● Withdraw your fingers.
● Discard the gloves, and wash your hands.

Performing a rectovaginal examination

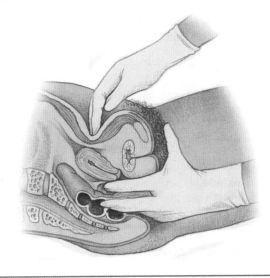

External male genitalia inspection

Penis

● Examine the skin, which should be slightly wrinkled and pink to light brown in white patients and light brown to dark brown in black patients.
● Check the penile shaft for lesions, nodules, inflammation, and swelling.
● Inspect the glans for discharge, genital warts, inflammation, lesions, swelling, and smegma (a cheesy secretion commonly found beneath the prepuce).
● Open the urethral meatus by gently compressing the tip of the glans.

Scrotum and testicles

● Ask the patient to hold his penis away from his scrotum.
● Observe the scrotum's size and appearance.
● Spread the surface of the scrotum and examine the skin for distended veins, nodules, redness, sebaceous cysts, swelling, and ulceration.

Inguinal and femoral areas

● Ask the patient to stand.
● Tell him to hold his breath and bear down while you inspect the inguinal and femoral areas for bulges and hernias.

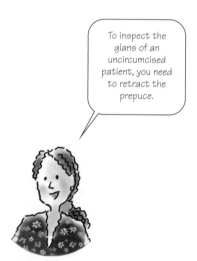

To inspect the glans of an uncircumcised patient, you need to retract the prepuce.

Examining the urethral meatus

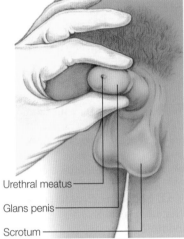

Urethral meatus

Glans penis

Scrotum

Penis and testicle palpation

Penis

- Use your thumb and forefinger to palpate the entire shaft of the penis.
  - The penis should be somewhat firm, with skin that's smooth and movable.
  - Note swelling, nodules, and indurations.

Testicles

- Gently palpate both testicles between your thumb and first two fingers.
  - The testicles should be equal in size; feel firm, smooth, and rubbery; and move freely in the scrotal sac.
- If you note hard, irregular areas or lumps, transilluminate them:
  - Darken the room.
  - Press the head of a flashlight against the scrotum, behind the lump.
  - Transilluminate the other testicle.
  - Compare your findings.
  - The testicles and any lumps, masses, warts, or blood-filled areas will appear as opaque shadows.
- Palpate the epididymides, which are located in the posterolateral area of the testicles.
  - They should be discrete, free from swelling and induration, nontender, and smooth.
- Palpate both spermatic cords, which are located above the testicles.
  - If you feel swelling, irregularity, or nodules, transilluminate the problem area.
  - If serous fluid is present, you won't see a glow.

Palpating the testes

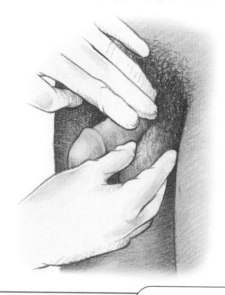

Your assessment of the testes offers you an opportunity to remind the patient to perform monthly self-testicular exams.

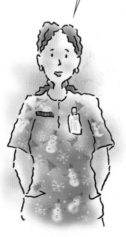

Inguinal hernia evaluation

- To assess for a direct inguinal hernia:
  - Place two fingers over each external inguinal ring.
  - Ask the patient to bear down.
  - If a hernia is present, you'll feel a bulge.
- To assess for an indirect inguinal hernia:
  - Examine the patient while he's standing; then examine him while he's supine, with his knee flexed on the side you're examining.
  - Place your index finger on the neck of the scrotum and gently push up into the inguinal canal.
  - Ask the patient to bear down or cough.
  - A hernia feels like a mass of tissue that withdraws when it meets the finger.

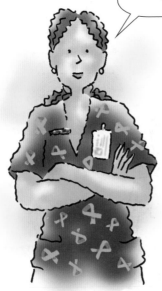

A direct inguinal hernia will feel like a bulge when the patient bears down. An indirect inguinal hernia will feel like a mass of tissue that withdraws as it meets the finger when he coughs or bears down.

Palpating for an indirect inguinal hernia

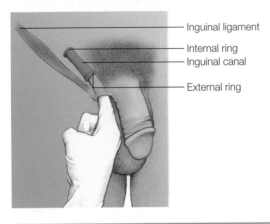

- Inguinal ligament
- Internal ring
- Inguinal canal
- External ring

Prostate gland palpation

● Have the patient stand and lean over the examination table.
● Lubricate the gloved index finger of your dominant hand.
● Insert your finger into the rectum.
● With your finger pad, palpate the prostate gland on the anterior rectal wall, just past the anorectal ring.
– It should feel smooth and rubbery.
– It should be about the size of a walnut. Enlargement classifications range from grade 1 (protruding less than $3/8''$ [1 cm] into the rectal lumen) to grade 4 (protruding more than $1\frac{1}{4}''$ [3.2 cm] into the rectal lumen).
– Ask the patient about tenderness.
– Note any nodules.

The prostate gland is normally about the size of a walnut.

Palpating the prostate gland

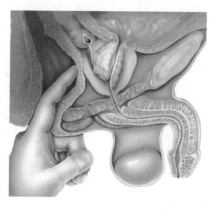

Vaginal abnormalities

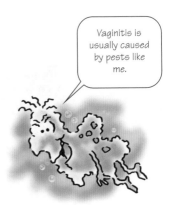

Vaginitis is usually caused by pests like me.

Vaginitis

- Usually results from an overgrowth of infectious organisms
- Causes redness, itching, dyspareunia (painful intercourse), dysuria, and a malodorous discharge
- Occurs with bacterial vaginosis, *Candida albicans* infection, trichomoniasis, and mucopurulent cervicitis

Candida albicans infection

- Produces a thick, white, curdlike discharge with a yeastlike odor
- Appears in patches on the cervix and vaginal walls

Mucopurulent cervicitis

- Produces purulent yellow discharge from the cervical os
- Occurs with trachomatis and gonorrhea

Trichomoniasis

- May produce a malodorous yellow or green, frothy or watery discharge
- May also cause red papules on the cervix and vaginal walls, giving the tissue a "strawberry" appearance

(Text continues on page 296.)

Looking at abnormal vaginal discharges

Vaginosis

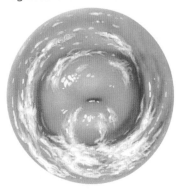

Candida albicans infection

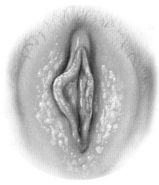

Mucopurulent cervicitis

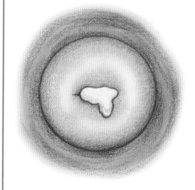

Trichomoniasis

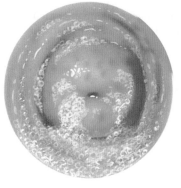

Vaginal abnormalities *(continued)*

Cervical polyps

● Characterized by bright red, soft, fragile nodules that usually arise from the endocervical canal and may bleed
● Typically benign

Cervical cancer

● Characterized by hard, granular, friable lesions (late stage)

Rectocele

● Occurs when the rectum herniates through the posterior vaginal wall
● On examination, presents as a pouch or bulging on the posterior vaginal wall as the patient bears down

Vaginal and uterine prolapse

● Also called *cystocele*
● Occurs when the anterior vaginal wall and bladder prolapse into the vagina
● During speculum examination, presents as a pouch or bulging on the anterior vaginal wall as the patient bears down

Recognizing genital abnormalities

Cervical polyps

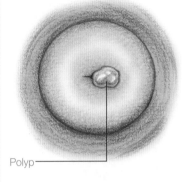

Polyp

Cervical cancer

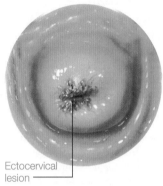

Ectocervical lesion

Rectocele

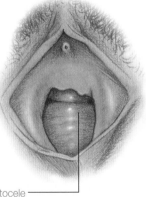

Rectocele

Vaginal and uterine prolapse

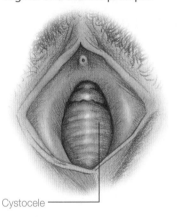

Cystocele

Sexually transmitted genital abnormalities

Syphilitic chancre

- In early stages, causes a red, painless, eroding lesion with a raised, indurated border; eventually erodes into an ulcer
- When palpated, may feel like a button
- In females, usually appears inside the vagina but may also appear on the external genitalia
- In males, appears on the surface of the penis

Genital warts

- Caused by the human papillomavirus
- Characterized by a flesh-colored, soft, moist, papillary growth that occurs singly or in cauliflower-like clusters
- May be barely visible or several inches in diameter
- May spontaneously resolve

Genital herpes

- Produces multiple, shallow vesicles, lesions, or crusts inside the vagina, on the external genitalia, on the buttocks, and sometimes on the thighs (in females) or on the prepuce, shaft, or glans (in males)
- May be accompanied by dysuria, regional lymph node inflammation, pain, edema, and fever
- Lesions eventually disappear but tend to recur

Identifying genital lesions of sexually transmitted diseases

Syphilitic chancre (female)

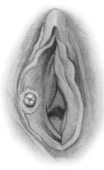

Syphilitic chancre (male)

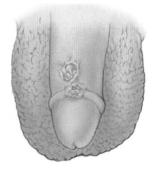

Genital warts (female)

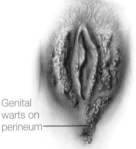

Genital warts on perineum

Genital warts (male)

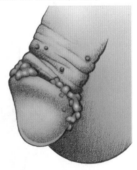

Genital herpes (female)

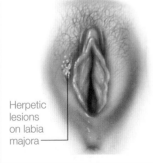

Herpetic lesions on labia majora

Genital herpes (male)

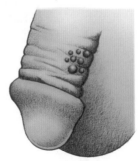

Male genital abnormalities

Penile cancer

- Causes a painless, ulcerative lesion on the glans or prepuce (foreskin)
- May be accompanied by discharge

Testicular tumor

- A painless scrotal nodule that can't be transilluminated
- May be benign or cancerous
- May grow, enlarging the testes

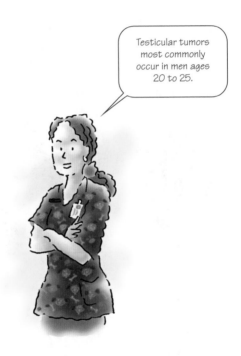

Testicular tumors most commonly occur in men ages 20 to 25.

Identifying penile and testicular cancer

Penile cancer

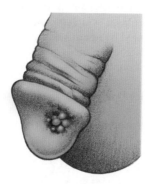

Testicular tumor

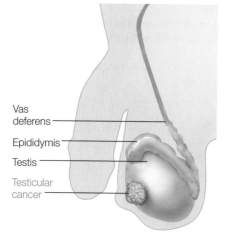

Vas deferens
Epididymis
Testis
Testicular cancer

Prostate abnormalities

Prostate gland enlargement

- Smooth, firm, symmetrical enlargement of the prostate gland indicates benign prostatic hyperplasia, which typically starts after age 50.
- Finding may be accompanied by nocturia, urinary hesitancy and frequency, recurring urinary tract infections, sensations of suprapubic fullness and incomplete bladder emptying, perineal pain, constipation, and hematuria.
- The patient may experience reduced force of and an inability to stop the urine stream.
- With acute prostatitis, the prostate gland is firm, warm, and extremely tender and swollen.

Prostate gland lesions

- Hard, irregular, and fixed lesions that make the prostate feel asymmetrical suggest prostate cancer.
- Palpation may be painful.
- The patient may also experience urinary dysfunction, such as urinary frequency, urinary urgency, or nocturia; perineal pain; constipation; fatigue; and weight loss.
- With cancerous lesions that metastasize to bone, back and leg pain may occur in advanced stages.

Identifying prostate gland enlargement and lesions

Prostate enlargement

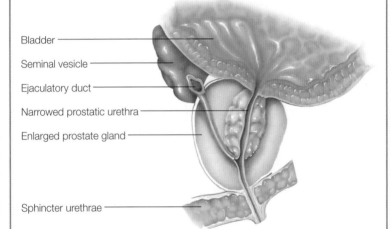

Bladder

Seminal vesicle

Ejaculatory duct

Narrowed prostatic urethra

Enlarged prostate gland

Sphincter urethrae

Prostate lesion

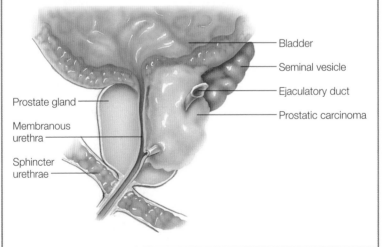

Bladder

Seminal vesicle

Ejaculatory duct

Prostatic carcinoma

Prostate gland

Membranous urethra

Sphincter urethrae

10

Breasts and axillae

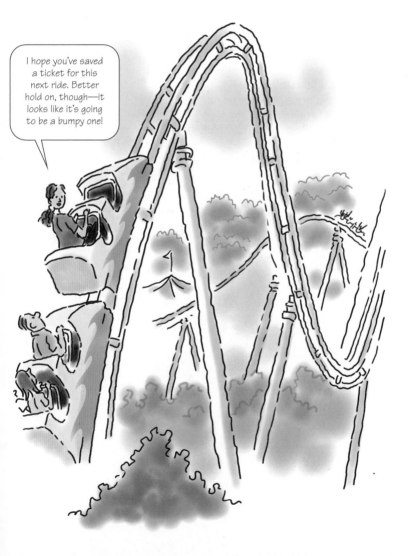

Breast inspection

● Ask the patient to disrobe from the waist up and sit with her arms at her side.
● The breast skin should be smooth, undimpled, and the same color as the rest of the skin.
● Check for edema, which can accompany lymphatic obstruction and may signal cancer.
● Inspect the nipples.
  – Note their size and shape.
  – If inverted (dimpled or creased), ask the patient when she first noticed the inversion.
● To detect skin or nipple dimpling that might not be obvious, inspect the breasts while the patient:
  – holds her arms over her head.
  – has her hands on her hips.
● If the patient has large or pendulous breasts, have her stand with her hands on the back of a chair and lean forward. This position helps reveal subtle breast and nipple asymmetry.

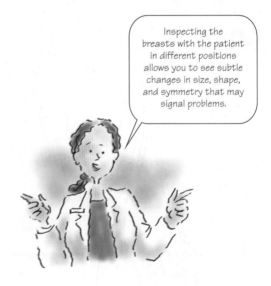

Inspecting the breasts with the patient in different positions allows you to see subtle changes in size, shape, and symmetry that may signal problems.

Inspecting the breasts

Arms at side

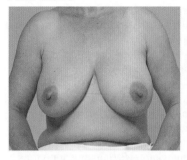

Arms overhead

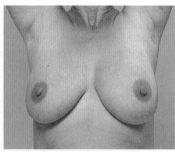

Hands pressed against hips

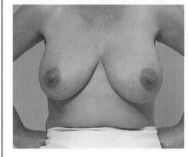

Leaning forward

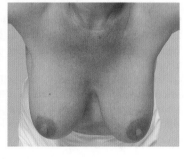

Breast development

● Observe breast size and shape, keeping in mind normal development throughout the life span:

– Before age 8: The breast and nipple area is flat.

– Ages 8 to 13: Development usually starts with the breast and nipple protruding as a single mound of flesh.

– Adolescence and adulthood: Breast size develops. Skin should be smooth and undimpled. Breasts may be symmetrical or asymmetrical.

– Adulthood (during pregnancy): Areolae become deeply pigmented and increase in diameter. The nipples become darker, more prominent, and erect. The breasts enlarge because of proliferation and hypertrophy of the alveolar cells and lactiferous ducts. As veins engorge, a venous pattern may become visible. Striae may appear as a result of stretching, and Montgomery's tubercles may become prominent.

– Adulthood (after pregnancy): During breast-feeding, the breasts become full and tense and may feel firm and warm. After breast-feeding ceases, breast size decreases but usually doesn't return to the prepregnancy state.

– Adulthood (after menopause): The breasts become flabbier and smaller. As the ligaments relax, the breasts hang loosely from the chest. The nipples flatten, losing some of their erectile quality. The ducts around the nipples may feel like firm strings.

As you perform your examination, remember that aging and pregnancy change the characteristics of the breasts.

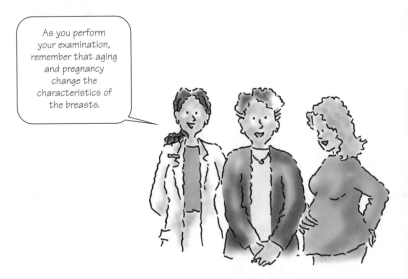

Identifying breast changes through the life span

Before age 8

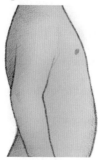

During pregnancy

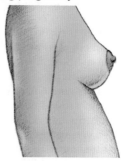

Between ages 8 and 13

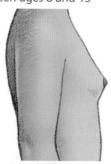

After pregnancy

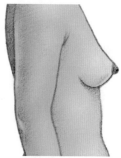

During adulthood
(having never given birth)

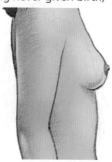

After menopause

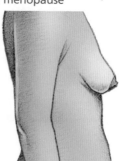

Breast palpation

● Use the pads of the fingertips, applying different amounts of pressure to examine different levels of the breast:
  – Apply light pressure to assess the area just underneath the skin.
  – Apply medium pressure to assess the tissue midway through the breast.
  – Apply deep pressure to assess the deepest tissue in the breast.
● Choose a method to palpate the breast:
  – Circular method: Move your fingers in a concentric circle around the entire breast.
  – Wedged method: Move your fingers outward from the nipple, making your way around the entire breast.
  – Vertical strip method: Move your fingers up and down over the breast in a vertical line.
● Be consistent and palpate the entire breast, including the periphery, tail of Spence, and areola.

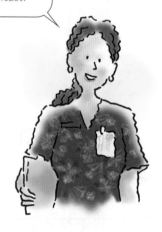

According to the American Cancer Society, the vertical strip method is the best way to ensure you've palpated the entire breast.

(Text continues on page 312.)

Looking at breast palpation methods

Circular

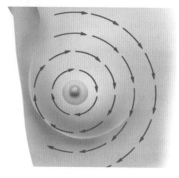

Wedged

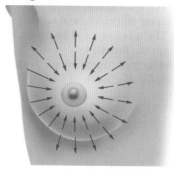

Vertical strip

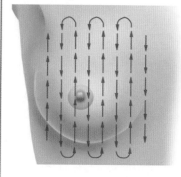

Breast palpation *(continued)*

- Ask the patient to lie in a supine position.
- Place a small pillow under the patient's shoulder on the side you're examining.
  - Doing so causes the breast on that side to protrude.
- Unless the patient's breasts are small, have the patient put her hand behind her head on the side you're examining.
  - This position spreads the breast more evenly across the chest and makes finding nodules easier.
- Use your three middle fingers to palpate the breast systematically.
- Rotate your fingers gently against the chest wall, moving in a consistent manner.
- Note the consistency of the breast tissue, keeping in mind that normal consistency varies widely, depending in part on the proportions of fat and glandular tissue.
- Check for nodules and unusual tenderness.
  - Tenderness may be related to cysts and cancer.
- Palpate the areola and nipple.
  - The nipple should be rough, elastic, and round and should protrude from the breast.
- Gently squeeze the nipple between your thumb and index finger to check for discharge.

Performing breast palpation

Examining the breast and axilla

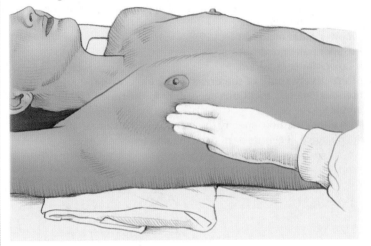

Examining the areola and breast

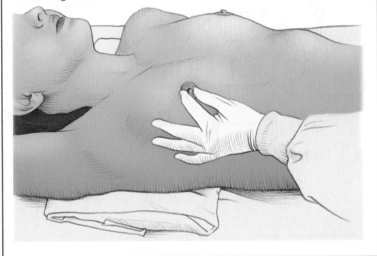

Breast lesion locations

● Mentally divide the breast into four quadrants and a fifth segment, the tail of Spence.
● Describe your findings according to the appropriate quadrant or segment:
  – Upper outer quadrant
  – Lower outer quadrant
  – Upper inner quadrant
  – Lower inner quadrant.
● Alternatively, think of the breast as a clock, with the nipple in the center, and specify locations according to the time (2 o'clock, for example).
● With either method, specify the location of a lesion or other findings by its distance in centimeters from the nipple.

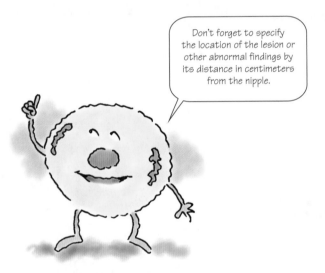

Don't forget to specify the location of the lesion or other abnormal findings by its distance in centimeters from the nipple.

Identifying locations of breast lesions

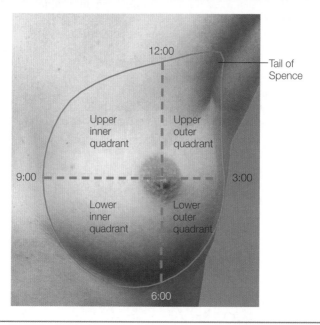

12:00

Tail of Spence

Upper inner quadrant

Upper outer quadrant

9:00

3:00

Lower inner quadrant

Lower outer quadrant

6:00

It's your choice! If you're good at geometry, use the quadrant method to describe the location of your findings. If you're good at telling time, use the clock method.

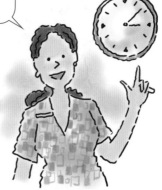

Breast lumps

● If you find a breast mass during your assessment, evaluate it using this flowchart.
● If you palpate a mass, record these characteristics:
  – size in centimeters
  – shape (round, discoid, regular, or irregular)
  – consistency (soft, firm, or hard)
  – degree of tenderness
  – location, using the quadrant or clock method.
● Note that masses may be further investigated with a biopsy.

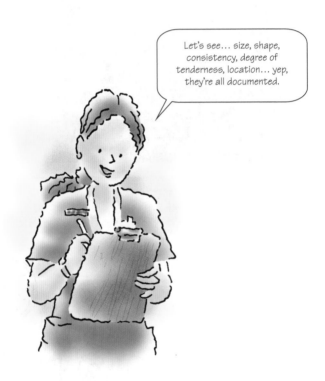

Let's see... size, shape, consistency, degree of tenderness, location... yep, they're all documented.

Evaluating a breast lump

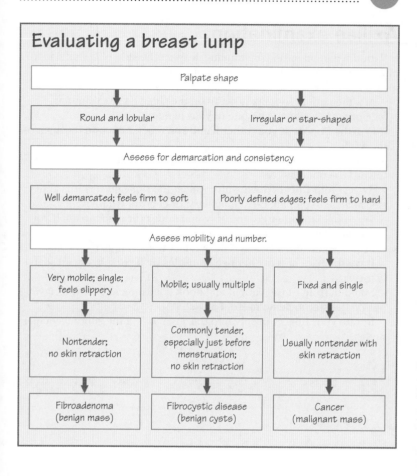

Axillae examination

● With the patient sitting or standing, inspect the skin of the axillae for rashes, infections, and unusual pigmentation.
● To palpate the axilla:
  – Ask the patient to relax her arm on the side you're examining.
  – Support her elbow with one of your hands.
  – Cup the fingers of your other hand, and reach high into the apex of the axilla.
  – Place your fingers directly behind the pectoral muscles, pointing toward the midclavicle.
  – Sweep your fingers downward against the ribs and serratus anterior muscle to palpate the midaxillary, or central, lymph nodes.
  – Try to palpate other groups of lymph nodes for comparison if you feel a hard, large, or tender lesion.
● Assess the clavicular nodes if the axillary nodes appear abnormal:
  – Have the patient relax her neck muscles by flexing her head slightly forward.
  – Stand in front of the patient and hook your fingers over the clavicle beside the sternocleidomastoid muscle.
  – Rotate your fingers deeply into this area to feel the supraclavicular nodes.

Palpating the axilla

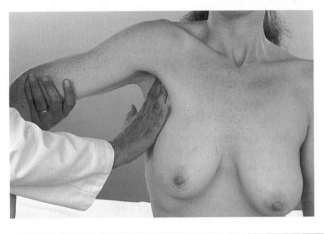

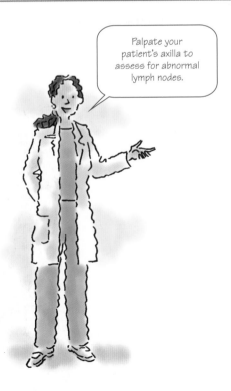

Palpate your patient's axilla to assess for abnormal lymph nodes.

Breast cancer

Breast cancer tumor

- Irregularly shaped mass with poorly defined edges on palpation
- Fixed mass that feels firm to hard and is usually nontender
- May cause skin retraction or nipple deviation or retraction
- May be accompanied by axillary lymphadenopathy
- Also may be accompanied by edema or peau d'orange of the skin overlying the mass

Ductal carcinoma in situ

- Earliest stage of development of breast cancer in which the abnormal cells remain confined to the ducts
- Also known as *intraductal carcinoma* or *noninvasive carcinoma*
- Most common type of carcinoma in situ in males and females

Infiltrating (invasive) ductal carcinoma

- Begins within the duct and spreads to the breast's parenchymal tissue
- May metastasize to other areas of the body.

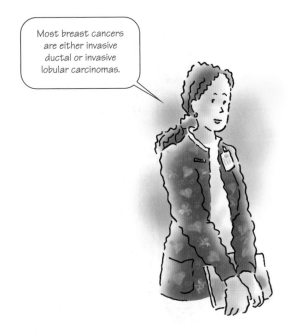

Most breast cancers are either invasive ductal or invasive lobular carcinomas.

Looking at breast cancer lesions

Breast cancer mass

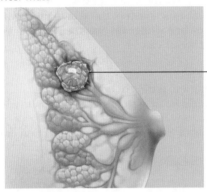

Irregular shape with poorly defined edges

Ductal carcinoma in situ

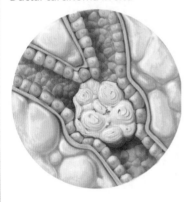

Infiltrating ductal carcinoma

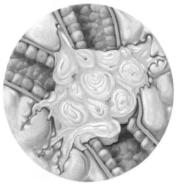

Breast abnormalities

Dimpling

- Puckering and retraction of the skin over the breast
- Results from abnormal attachment of the skin to underlying tissue
- Suggests inflammation or a malignant mass beneath the skin surface
- Usually a late sign of breast cancer

Peau d'orange

- Edematous thickening and pitting of breast skin
- Striking orange-peel appearance stems from lymphatic edema around deepened hair follicles
- May occur with breast or axillary lymph node infection or Grave's disease
- Usually a late sign of breast cancer

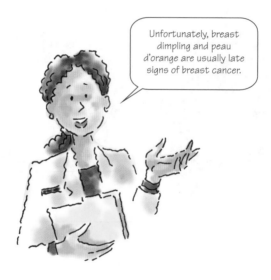

Unfortunately, breast dimpling and peau d'orange are usually late signs of breast cancer.

Identifying dimpling and peau d'orange

Dimpling

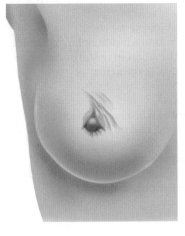

Peau d'orange

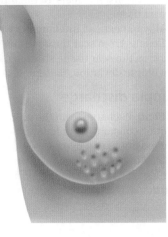

Nipple abnormalities

Nipple retraction

- Inward displacement of the nipple below the level of the surrounding breast tissue
- May indicate an inflammatory breast lesion or cancer
- Results from scar tissue formation within a lesion or large mammary duct; as the scar tissue shortens, it pulls adjacent tissue inward, causing nipple deviation, flattening, and, finally, retraction

Nipple discharge

- Fluid discharge from the nipple that can be characterized as intermittent or constant, as unilateral or bilateral, and by color, consistency, composition, and odor
- May occur spontaneously or by nipple stimulation
- May be a normal finding or may signal serious underlying disease, particularly when accompanied by other breast changes

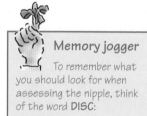

Memory jogger

To remember what you should look for when assessing the nipple, think of the word DISC:

Discharge

Inversion

Skin changes

Contrast (to other side).

Looking at nipple retraction

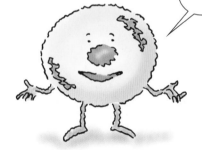

Nipple retraction occurs when scar tissue shortens and pulls adjacent tissue inward, flattening and displacing the nipple at the surface. It may be an indication of an inflammatory breast lesion or cancer.

Fibrotic changes

Fibrocystic changes

- Also known as *benign cysts*
- Round, elastic, mobile masses that are commonly tender on palpation, especially around menstruation
- May include multiple cysts
- May be accompanied by clear, watery (serous) discharge or a sticky nipple
- Typically not accompanied by skin retraction

Fibroadenoma

- Benign, round, lobular, and well-demarcated mobile mass that feels slippery and firm to soft on palpation
- Usually nontender
- Usually located around the nipple or on the lateral side of the upper outer quadrant
- Typically not accompanied by skin retraction

Looking at fibrotic changes

Fibrocystic changes

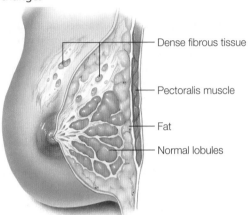

Dense fibrous tissue

Pectoralis muscle

Fat

Normal lobules

Fibroadenoma

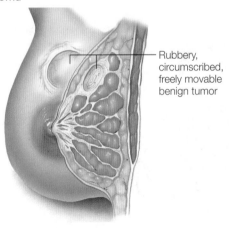

Rubbery, circumscribed, freely movable benign tumor

Mastitis and breast engorgement

- Disorders that affect lactating females

Mastitis

- Develops when a pathogen in the breast-feeding infant's nose or oropharynx invades breast tissue through a fissured or cracked nipple and disrupts normal lactation
- Characterized by a tender, hard, swollen, and warm breast
- May be accompanied by flulike signs and symptoms, including fever, malaise, fatigue, and body aches

Breast engorgement

- Results from venous and lymphatic stasis and alveolar milk accumulation
- Causes painful breasts that feel heavy and possibly warm

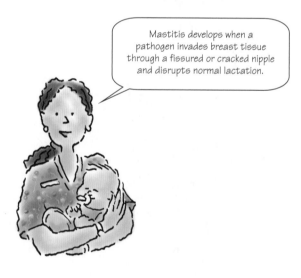

Mastitis develops when a pathogen invades breast tissue through a fissured or cracked nipple and disrupts normal lactation.

Identifying mastitis and breast engorgement

Mastitis

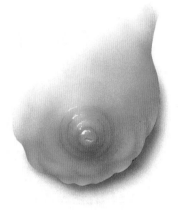

Breast engorgement

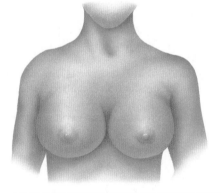

Male breast abnormalities

- Examine a man's breasts thoroughly during a complete physical assessment.
- Assess for the same changes you would assess for in a woman.

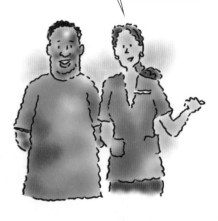

Remember that men can also experience breast abnormalities.

Breast cancer

- Usually occurs in the areolar area
- Is invasive ductal carcinoma in 80% to 90% of cases

Gynecomastia

- Abnormal enlargement of the male breast
- Usually caused by a disklike growth under the nipple
- Most common male breast disorder
- May be barely palpable and is usually bilateral
- Can be caused by cirrhosis, leukemia, thyrotoxicosis, hormones, illicit drug use, or alcohol consumption
- In adolescent boys:
  - temporary stimulation of breast tissue is caused by estrogen
  - adequate testosterone production usually ceases enlargement.
- In elderly men:
  - age-related hormonal alterations and certain medications can cause enlargement.

Identifying gynecomastia

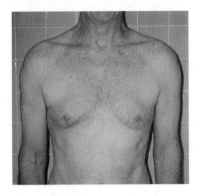

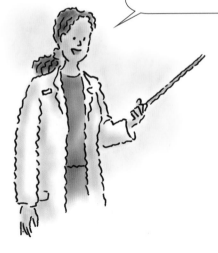

Gynecomastia is usually bilateral and may be barely palpable. It's the most common male breast disorder.

11

Musculoskeletal system

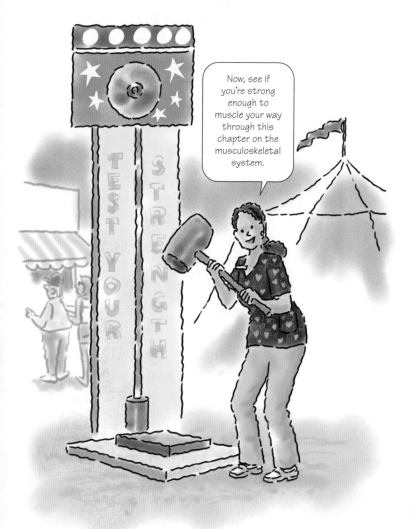

Bone and joint assessment

● Begin with a general observation of your patient, checking for general symmetry. Whenever possible, observe how the patient stands and moves.

● Note the size and shape of joints, limbs, and body regions.

● Systematically assess the whole body, working from head to toe and from proximal to distal structures.

● Because muscles and joints are interdependent, interpret these findings together.

● Have the patient perform active range-of-motion (ROM) exercises, if possible.

● If he can't perform active ROM exercises, perform passive ROM exercises:

  – Support the joint firmly on either side.
  – Move the joint gently to avoid causing pain or spasm.
  – Never force movement.

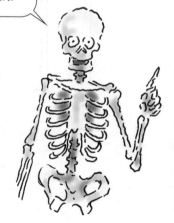

Active ROM exercises are joint movements the patient can do without assistance. Passive ROM exercises don't require the patient to exert effort.

Understanding types of joint movement

Retraction and protraction
Moving backward and forward

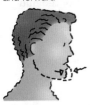

Flexion
Bending, decreasing the joint angle

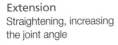

Extension
Straightening, increasing the joint angle

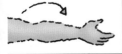

Circumduction
Moving in a circular manner

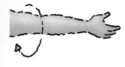

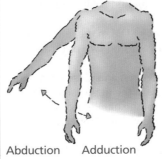
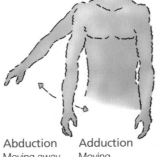

Abduction
Moving away from midline

Adduction
Moving toward midline

Internal rotation
Turning toward midline

External rotation
Turning away from midline

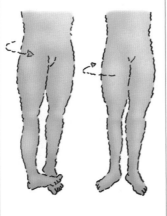

Supination
Turning upward

Pronation
Turning downward

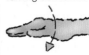

Eversion
Turning outward

Inversion
Turning inward

Head and jaw assessment

● Inspect the patient's face for swelling, symmetry, and evidence of trauma. The mandible should be at the midline, not shifted to the right or left.

● Evaluate the patient's ROM in the temporomandibular joint (TMJ):

– Place the tips of your first two or three fingers in front of the middle of the ear.

– Ask the patient to open and close his mouth.

– Place your fingers in the depressed area over the joint.

– Note the motion of the mandible. The patient should be able to open and close the jaw and protract and retract the mandible easily, without pain or tenderness.

– If you hear or palpate a click as the patient's mouth opens, suspect an improperly aligned jaw.

– Note whether TMJ dysfunction is accompanied by swelling, crepitus (abnormal grating sound), or pain.

Evaluating the temporomandibular joint

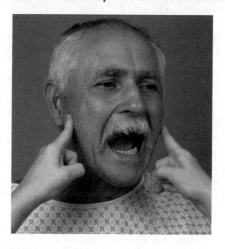

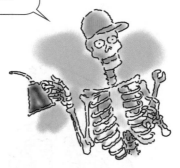

TMJ dysfunction may be accompanied by swelling, pain, and crepitus—an abnormal grating sound that gets on my last nerve!

Neck assessment

- Inspect the front, back, and sides of the patient's neck, noting muscle asymmetry and masses.
- Palpate the spinous processes of the cervical vertebrae and the areas above each clavicle (supraventricular fossae) for tenderness, swelling, and nodules:
  - Stand facing the patient with your hands placed lightly on the sides of his neck.
  - Ask him to turn his head from side to side, flex his neck forward, and then extend it backward.
  - Feel for lumps and tender areas.
  - Listen and palpate for crepitus as the patient moves his neck.
- Check ROM in the neck:
  - Ask the patient to try touching his right ear to his right shoulder and his left ear to his left shoulder. Typical ROM is 40 degrees on each side.
  - Ask the patient to touch his chin to his chest and then to point this chin up toward the ceiling. The neck should flex forward 45 degrees and extend backward 55 degrees.
  - Assess rotation by asking the patient to turn his head to each side without moving his trunk. The chin should be parallel to the shoulders.
  - Ask the patient to move his head in a circle. Normal rotation is 70 degrees.

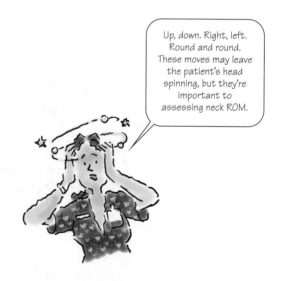

Up, down. Right, left. Round and round. These moves may leave the patient's head spinning, but they're important to assessing neck ROM.

Assessing neck range of motion

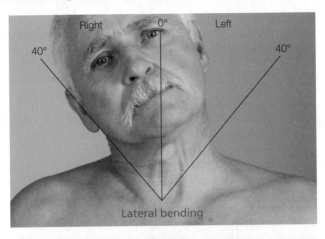

Right   0°   Left

40°   40°

Lateral bending

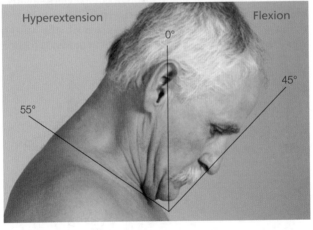

Hyperextension   Flexion

0°

55°   45°

Spinal assessment

● Assess spinal position and curvature as the patient stands in profile. The spine should have a reverse "S" shape.

● Observe the spine posteriorly. It should be midline in position, without deviation to either side.

● Palpate the spinal processes and the areas lateral to the spine:
   – Have the patient bend at the waist and let his arms hang loosely at his sides.
   – Palpate the spine with your fingertips.
   – Repeat the palpation using the side of your hand, lightly striking the areas lateral to the spine.
   – Note tenderness, swelling, or spasm.

● Assess the range of spinal movement:
   – Ask the patient to straighten up.
   – Use a measuring tape to determine the distance from the nape of the neck to the waist.
   – Ask the patient to bend forward at the waist, continuing to hold the tape at his neck and letting it slip through your fingers slightly to accommodate the increased distance as the spine flexes.
   – Note that the length of the spine from the neck to the waist usually increases by at least 2″ (5.1 cm) when the patient bends forward.

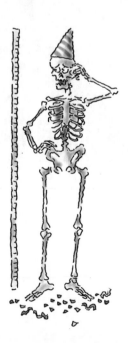

So let me get this straight… If I lean forward and bend from the waist, I'm technically taller than if I stand upright to be measured?

Assessing the range of spinal movement

Standing straight up

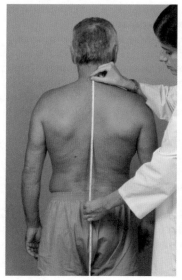

Bending over

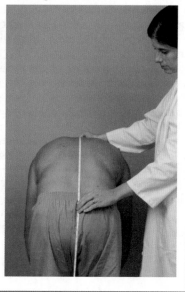

Shoulder assessment

- Observe the patient's shoulders. Note asymmetry, muscle atrophy, or deformity.
- Palpate the shoulders with the palmar surfaces of your fingers to locate bony prominences. Note crepitus or tenderness.
- Using your entire hand, palpate the shoulder muscles for firmness and symmetry.
- To assess abduction, ask the patient to move his arm from the neutral position laterally as far as possible. Normal ROM is 180 degrees.
- To assess adduction, ask the patient to move his arm from the neutral position across the front of his body as far as possible. Normal ROM is 50 degrees.
- To assess flexion, ask the patient to move his arm anteriorly from his side over his head. Full flexion is 180 degrees.
- To assess extension, ask him to move his arm from the neutral position posteriorly as far as possible. Normal extension ranges from 30 to 50 degrees.
- To assess external and internal rotation, ask the patient to adduct his arm with his elbow bent. Then ask him to place his fist behind the small of his back. Normal external and internal rotation is 90 degrees.

Assessing shoulder range of motion

Abduction and adduction

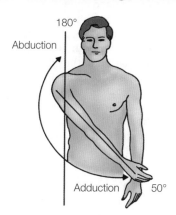

180°

Abduction

Adduction 50°

Flexion and extension

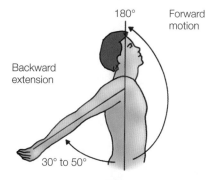

180° Forward motion

Backward extension

30° to 50°

External and internal rotation

90°

External rotation

Internal rotation

90°

Elbow assessment

- Assess the elbows for flexion and extension:
  - Have the patient rest his arm at his side.
  - Ask him to flex his elbow from this position and then extend it.
  - Normal ROM is 90 degrees for both flexion and extension.
- Assess supination and pronation of the elbow:
  - Have the patient place the sides of his hand on a flat surface with his thumb on top.
  - Ask him to rotate his palm down toward the table for pronation and upward for supination.
  - Normal angle of elbow rotation is 90 degrees in each direction.

Assessing elbow range of motion

Flexion and extension

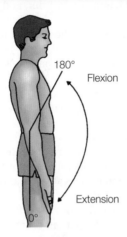

180°

Flexion

Extension

0°

Pronation and supination

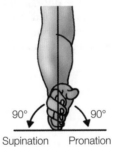

90°   90°

Supination   Pronation

Wrist and hand assessment

- Inspect the wrists and hands for contour, and compare them for symmetry.
- Check for nodules, redness, swelling, deformities, and webbing between fingers.
- Use your thumb and index finger to palpate both wrists and each finger joint.
    - Note tenderness or bogginess.
    - To avoid causing pain, be especially gentle with older adults and those with arthritis.
- Assess radial and ulnar deviation.
    - Ask the patient to rotate each wrist by moving his entire hand—first laterally, then medially—as if he were waxing a car.
    - Normal ROM is 55 degrees laterally (ulnar deviation) and 20 degrees medially (radial deviation).
- Assess wrist extension and flexion.
    - Observe the wrist while the patient extends his fingers up toward the ceiling and down toward the floor, as if he's flapping his hand. He should be able to extend his wrist 70 degrees and flex it 90 degrees.
    - If these movements cause pain or numbness, carpal tunnel syndrome may be present. Further assessment is needed.

Assessing wrist range of motion

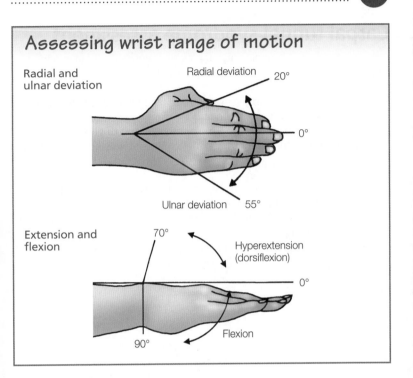

Radial and ulnar deviation

Radial deviation 20°

0°

Ulnar deviation 55°

Extension and flexion

70°

Hyperextension (dorsiflexion)

0°

90°

Flexion

Carpal tunnel syndrome assessment

- Assess for carpal tunnel syndrome by testing for Tinel's sign and Phalen's sign.
- Tinel's sign:
    - Lightly percuss the transverse carpal ligament over the median nerve where the patient's palm and wrist meet.
    - If this action produces shooting numbness and tingling into the palm and finger, the patient has Tinel's sign and may have carpal tunnel syndrome.
- Phalen's sign:
    - Have the patient put the backs of his hands together and flex his wrists downward at a 90-degree angle.
    - Pain or numbness in the hand or fingers during this maneuver indicates a positive Phalen's sign.
    - The more severe the carpal tunnel syndrome, the more rapidly symptoms develop.

Pressure on the median nerve produces the numbness, pain, and hand weakness that characterize carpal tunnel syndrome.

Testing for carpal tunnel syndrome

Tinel's sign

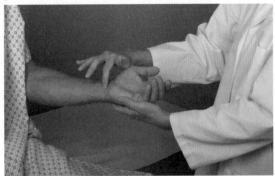

Phalen's sign

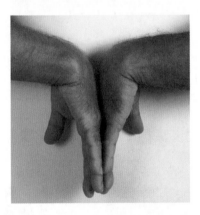

Finger assessment

- Assess extension and flexion of the metacarpophalangeal joints:
  - Ask the patient to keep his wrist still and move only his fingers—first up toward the ceiling and then down toward the floor.
  - Have the patient make a fist with his thumb remaining straight. Normal extension is 30 degrees; normal flexion is 90 degrees.
  - Ask the patient to touch the thumb of one hand to the little finger of the same hand.
  - He should be able to fold or flex his thumb across the palm of his hand so that it touches or points toward the base of his little finger.
- Assess flexion of all the fingers:
  - Ask the patient to form a fist.
  - Have him spread his fingers apart to demonstrate abduction and draw them back to demonstrate adduction.

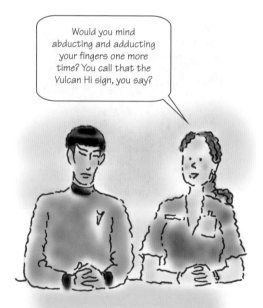

Would you mind abducting and adducting your fingers one more time? You call that the Vulcan Hi sign, you say?

Assessing finger range of motion

Extension and flexion

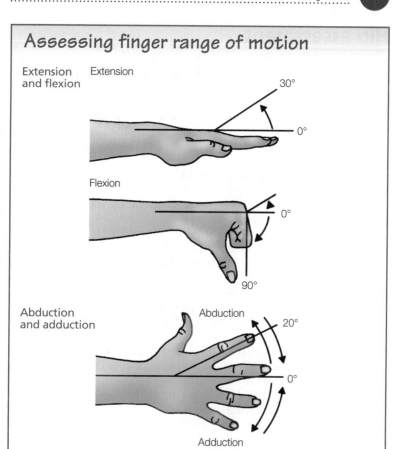

Extension

30°
0°

Flexion

0°
90°

Abduction and adduction

Abduction
20°
0°
Adduction

Hip assessment

- Inspect the hip area for contour and symmetry.
- Palpate each hip over the iliac crest and trochanteric area for tenderness or instability.
- Assess flexion of the hip:
  - Ask the patient to lie on his back and then bend one knee and pull it toward his abdomen and chest as far as possible.
  - As the patient flexes his knee, the opposite hip and thigh should remain flat.
  - Repeat the test on the opposite side.
- Assess extension of the hip:
  - Ask the patient to lie in a prone position (facedown) and gently extend the thigh upward.
  - Repeat the test on the other side.
- Assess internal and external rotation of the hip:
  - Ask the patient to bend his knee and turn his leg inward; then ask him to turn his leg outward.
- Assess hip abduction and adduction:
  - Stand alongside the patient at hip level.
  - Press down on the superior iliac spine of the opposite hip with one hand to stabilize the pelvis.
  - With your other hand, hold the patient's leg by the ankle and gently abduct the hip until you feel the iliac spine move. That movement indicates the limit of hip abduction.
  - While stabilizing the pelvis, move the ankle medially across the patient's body to assess hip adduction.
  - Repeat the procedure on the other side.

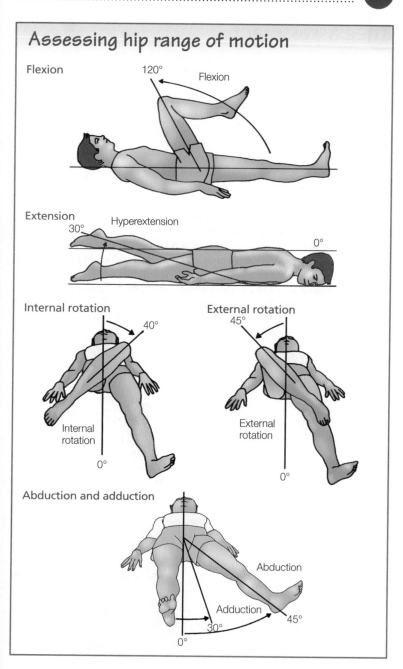

Assessing hip range of motion

Flexion

Flexion 120°

Extension

30° Hyperextension 0°

Internal rotation

40°

Internal rotation

0°

External rotation

45°

External rotation

0°

Abduction and adduction

Abduction

Adduction

45°

30°

0°

Knee assessment

● Inspect the position of the patient's knees, noting whether he has bowlegs (knees that point out laterally) or knock-knees (knees that turn in medially).

● Palpate both knees. They should feel smooth and the tissues should feel solid.

● Assess knee ROM:
  – If the patient is standing, ask him to bend his knee as if trying to touch his heel to his buttocks. Normal ROM is 120 to 130 degrees.
  – If the patient is lying down, have him draw his knee up to his chest. His calf should touch his thigh.

● Assess for bulge sign:
  – Ask the patient to lie down with his knee extended.
  – Place your left hand above the knee.
  – Apply pressure to the suprapatellar pouch to displace the fluid downward, or stroke downward on the medial aspect of the knee and apply pressure to force the fluid to the lateral area.
  – Tap the knee just behind the lateral margin of the patella.
  – Watch for a fluid wave—a positive bulge sign.

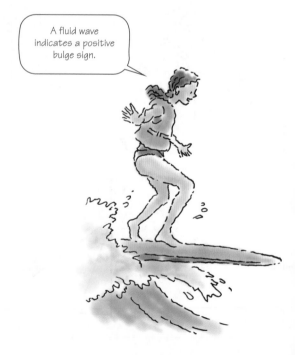

A fluid wave indicates a positive bulge sign.

Assessing knee range of motion

Flexion and extension

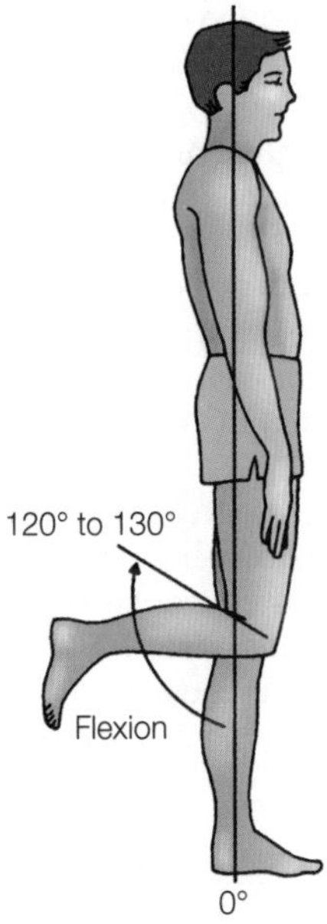

120° to 130°

Flexion

0°

Ankle and foot assessment

- Inspect the ankles and feet for swelling, redness, nodules, and other deformities.
- Check the arch of each foot and look for toe deformities. Note calluses, bunions, corns, ingrown toenails, plantar warts, trophic ulcers, hair loss, or unusual pigmentation.
- Use your fingertips to palpate the bony and muscular structures of the ankles and feet. Palpate each toe joint by compressing it with your thumb and fingers.
- Assess ROM of the ankles and feet:
  - Ask the patient to sit in a chair or on the side of the bed.
  - Test plantar flexion of the ankle by asking the patient to bend his ankle towards the floor. Normal ROM for plantar flexion is about 45 degrees.
  - Test dorsiflexion by asking him to bend his ankle towards the ceiling. Normal ROM for dorsiflexion is about 20 degrees.
  - Ask the patient to demonstrate inversion by turning his feet inward and eversion by turning his feet outward. Normal ROM for inversion is 30 degrees; for eversion, 20 degrees.
  - Assess the metatarsophalangeal joints by asking the patient to flex his toes and then straighten them.

Assessing ankle and foot range of motion

Plantar flexion and dorsiflexion

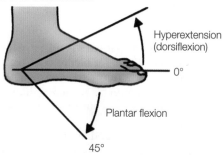

Hyperextension (dorsiflexion)

0°

Plantar flexion

45°

Eversion and inversion

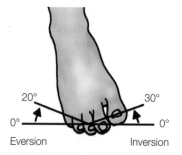

20°   30°

0°   0°

Eversion   Inversion

Muscle strength assessment

- Inspect all major muscle groups, checking for symmetry.
- Ask the patient to attempt normal ROM against your resistance. If the muscle group is weak, vary the amount of resistance as required to permit accurate measurement.

Arm muscles

- Biceps: With your hand on the patient's hand, have him flex his forearm against your resistance. Watch for biceps contractions.
- Deltoid: With the patient's arm fully extended, place one hand over his deltoid muscle and the other on his wrist. Ask him to abduct his arm to a horizontal position against your resistance; as he does so, palpate for deltoid contraction.
- Triceps: Have the patient abduct and hold his arm midway between flexion and extension. Hold and support his arm at the wrist and ask him to extend it against your resistance. Watch for triceps contraction.
- Dorsal interosseal: Have the patient extend and spread his fingers. Then tell him to try to resist your attempt to squeeze them.
- Forearm and hand (grip): Ask the patient to grasp your middle and index fingers and squeeze as hard as he can. Cross your fingers during this test to prevent injury.

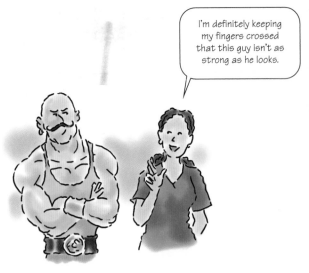

I'm definitely keeping my fingers crossed that this guy isn't as strong as he looks.

(Text continues on page 360.)

Testing arm muscle strength

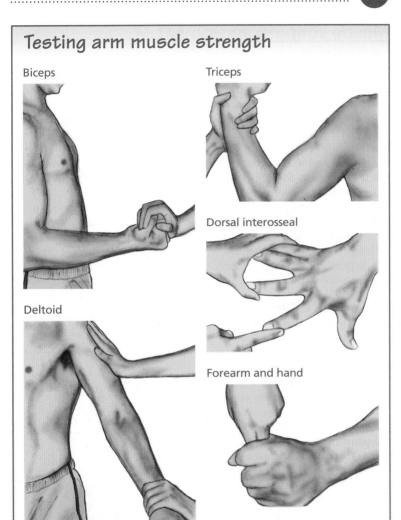

Biceps

Triceps

Dorsal interosseal

Deltoid

Forearm and hand

Muscle strength assessment *(continued)*

Leg muscles

● Anterior tibial: With the patient's leg extended, place your hand on his foot and ask him to dorsiflex his ankle against your resistance. Palpate for anterior tibial contraction.

● Psoas: While you support the patient's leg, ask the patient to raise his knee and then flex his hip against your resistance. Watch for psoas contraction.

● Extensor hallucis longus: With your finger on the patient's great toe, ask the patient to dorsiflex the toe against your resistance. Palpate for extensor hallucis contraction.

● Quadriceps: Have the patient bend his knee slightly while you support his lower leg. Then ask him to extend the knee against your resistance; as he's doing so, palpate for quadriceps contraction.

● Gastrocnemius: With the patient on his side, support his foot and ask him to plantar-flex his ankle against your resistance. Palpate for gastrocnemius contraction.

Grading strength

● Grade muscle strength on a scale of 0 to 5:
   – 0/5: Zero = Total paralysis
   – 1/5: Trace = Visible or palpable contraction, but no movement
   – 2/5: Poor = Full muscle movement with the force of gravity eliminated
   – 3/5: Fair = Full muscle movement against gravity, but no movement against resistance
   – 4/5: Good = Full muscle movement against gravity, with partial movement against resistance
   – 5/5: Normal = Full muscle movement against gravity and resistance

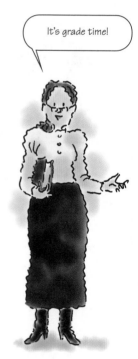

It's grade time!

Testing leg muscle strength

Anterior tibial

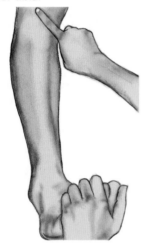

Psoas

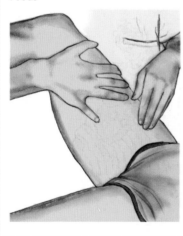

Extensor hallucis longus

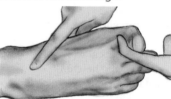

Quadriceps

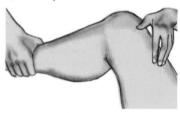

Gastrocnemius

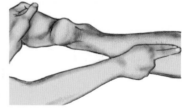

Scoliosis

- Lateral deviation of the spine that causes the patient to lean to one side
- May cause:
  - uneven shoulder blade height and shoulder blade prominence
  - unequal distance between the arms and the body
  - asymmetrical waist
  - uneven hip height
  - asymmetrical thoracic spine or prominent rib cage (rib hump) on either side
- May be caused by diskitis or spondylolisthesis

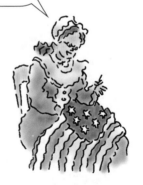

Lateral deviation that causes a person to lean to one side... I thought that was the definition of a conservative, or a liberal, for that matter. I didn't know it meant scoliosis, too!

Identifying scoliosis

Standing straight

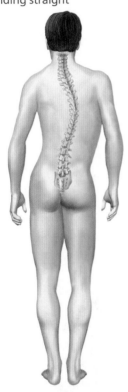

Bending over

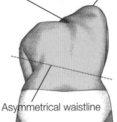

Asymmetrical thoracic spine

Rib hump

Asymmetrical waistline

Kyphosis and lordosis

Kyphosis

- Abnormally rounded thoracic curve
- Leads to hunchback or slouching posture
- May be caused by trauma, osteoporosis, degenerative joint disease, or developmental disorders
- May occur with scoliosis

Lordosis

- Abnormally concave lumbar spine
- Normal in pregnant women and young children
- Also called *swayback*

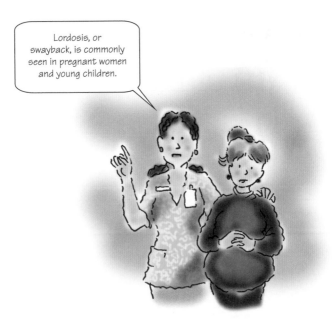

Lordosis, or swayback, is commonly seen in pregnant women and young children.

Identifying kyphosis and lordosis

Kyphosis

Lordosis

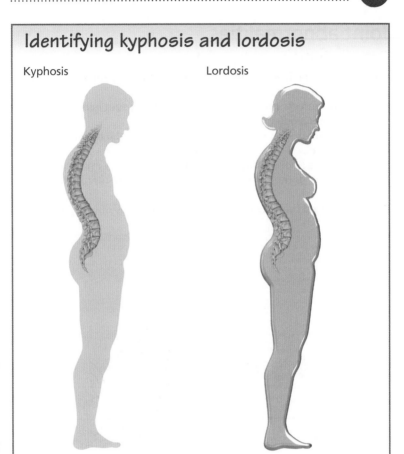

Joint abnormalities

Osteoarthritis

- Breakdown and loss of joint cartilage that causes pain in the joint, especially after repetitive use
- Commonly affects the hands, feet, spine, knees, and hips
- May be accompanied by:
  - Heberden's nodes: Hard, bony, cartilaginous enlargements that appear on the distal interphalangeal joints
  - Bouchard's nodes: Bony outgrowths or gelatinous cysts caused by calcific spurs of the joint cartilage of the proximal interphalangeal joints
- Mostly caused by aging but may also be caused by obesity, trauma, or surgery

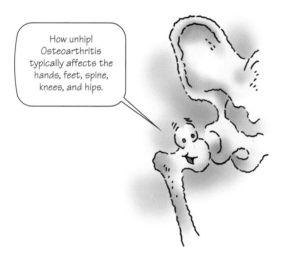

How unhip! Osteoarthritis typically affects the hands, feet, spine, knees, and hips.

(Text continues on page 368.)

Recognizing Heberden's and Bouchard's nodes

Heberden's nodes

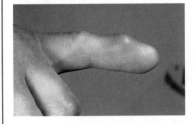

Bouchard's nodes

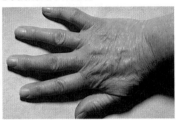

Heberden's and Bouchard's nodes may be red, swollen, and painful initially. But eventually, they become painless and can limit joint mobility.

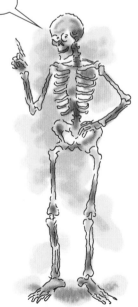

Joint abnormalities *(continued)*
Rheumatoid arthritis

- Chronic, systemic, inflammatory immune disorder
- Characterized by swollen, painful, and stiff joints
- Commonly affects the bilateral joints of the fingers, wrists, elbows, knees, and ankles as well as surrounding muscles, tendons, ligaments, and blood vessels
- May have spontaneous remissions and unpredictable exacerbations
- Leads to bone atrophy and misalignment that cause visible deformities, restriction of movement, and muscle atrophy
- May cause:
  - Swan-neck deformity: Hyperextension of the proximal interphalangeal joints with flexion of the distal interphalangeal joints
  - Boutonnière deformity: Flexion of the proximal interphalangeal joints with hyperextension of the distal interphalangeal joints

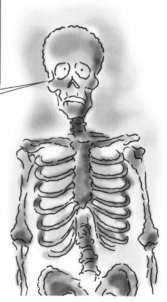

Rheumatoid arthritis affects not only the joints of the fingers, wrists, elbows, knees, and ankles, but also the surrounding muscles, tendons, ligaments, and blood vessels. I think I'd better inventory what it doesn't affect!

(Text continues on page 370.)

Looking at acute and chronic rheumatoid arthritis

Acute rheumatoid arthritis

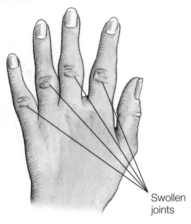

Swollen joints

Chronic rheumatoid arthritis

Boutonnière deformity

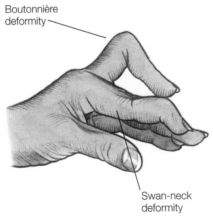

Swan-neck deformity

Joint abnormalities *(continued)*
Gout

● Metabolic disorder in which uric acid deposits in the joints
● Usually affects the joint of the big toe
● Causes joints to become painful, arthritic, red, and swollen, with attacks typically being acute and occurring at night
● May elevate skin temperature due to irritation and inflammation

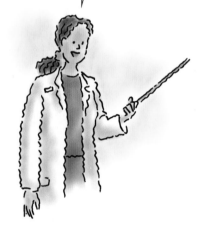

Risk factors for gout include hypertension, diabetes mellitus, hyperlipidemia, and arteriosclerosis.

Looking at gout

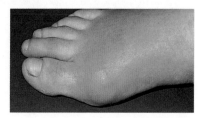

Credits

Herpes simplex, Angioedema, page 97. From Neville, B., et al. *Color Atlas of Clinical Pathology.* Philadelphia: Lea & Febiger, 1991.

Tonsillitis, Pharyngitis, page 101. Wellcome Photo Library.

Ahn, C., and Salcido, R. "Advances in Wound Photography and Assessment Methods," *Advances in Skin and Wound Care* 21(2): 85-93, February 2008.

Assessment: An Incredibly Easy! Pocket Guide. Philadelphia: Lippincott Williams & Wilkins, 2006.

Assessment. Lippincott Manual of Nursing Practice Series. Philadelphia: Lippincott Williams & Wilkins, 2007.

Assessment Made Incredibly Easy!, 4th ed. Philadelphia: Lippincott Williams & Wilkins, 2008.

Bickley, L.S., and Szilagyi, P.G. *Bates' Guide to Physical Examination and History Taking*, 9th ed. Philadelphia: Lippincott Williams & Wilkins, 2007.

Bonham, P., and Kelechi, T. "Evaluation of Lower Extremity Arterial Circulation and Implications for Nursing Practice," *Journal of Cardiovascular Nursing* 23(2): 144-52, March/April 2008.

Health Assessment Made Incredibly Visual! Philadelphia: Lippincott Williams & Wilkins, 2007.

Horgas, A., and Miller, L. "Pain Assessment in People with Dementia," *American Journal of Nursing* 108(7):62-70, July 2008.

Hunter, J., et al. "Respiratory Assessment," *Nursing Standards* 22(41):41-3, June 2008.

Jarvis, C. *Physical Assessment & Examination*, 5th ed. St. Louis: W.B. Saunders, 2008.

INDEX

Note: i refers to an illustration; t refers to a table.

A

Abdomen
  auscultating, 232, 233i
  identifying quadrants and structures of, 231i
  inspecting, 230
  palpating, 240, 241i
  percussing, 234, 235i
Abdominal aorta
  assessing, 248
  identifying, 249i
Abdominal distention, 258
  identifying, 259i
Abdominal pain, 260
  assessment of, 250, 251i, 252, 253i, 254, 255i
  identifying origins of, 262-263t
  types and causes of, 261t
Abdominal reflexes, testing, 142
Abdominal sounds
  abnormal, 264, 265t
  locations of, 233i, 265t
  normal, 234
Abducens nerve, 117i, 120, 121i
Achilles reflex, testing, 140, 141i
Acoustic nerve, 117i, 124
Actinic keratosis, precancerous, 30, 31i
Acute angle-closure glaucoma, 66, 67i
Adventitious breath sounds, 186, 187i, 188, 189i
Alopecia, 40, 41i
Anal examination. See Rectal and anal examination.
Angioedema, 96, 97i
Ankle assessment, 356, 357i
Aortic insufficiency, murmur in, 224, 225i
Aortic stenosis, murmur in, 224, 225i
Aphasia
  areas of the brain affected by, 149i
  types of, 148
Apical impulse, palpating, 194, 195i
Apnea, 182, 183i
Arterial insufficiency, 210, 211i
Arterial pulses
  grading, 204
  palpating, 204, 205i, 206, 207i
Arterial ulcers, 226, 227i
Ascites, assessing for, 246, 247i
Assessment
  recording initial findings of, 16, 17i
  techniques for, 8, 9i, 10, 11i, 12, 13i, 14, 15i

Auscultation as assessment technique, 14, 15i
Axillae
  inspecting, 318
  palpating, 313i, 318, 319i

B

Babinski's reflex, 142, 143i
Balance, testing, 136, 137i
Barrel chest, 178, 179i
Bartholin's glands, palpating, 274, 275i
Basal cell carcinoma, 30, 31i
Biceps reflex, testing, 138, 139i
Bimanual pelvic examination, 282, 283i
Biot's respirations, 184, 185i
Blood pressure measurement, 6, 7i
Bone assessment, 334
Bowel sounds, abnormal, 264, 265t
Brachial pulse, palpating, 204, 205i
Brachioradialis reflex, testing, 138, 139i
Bradypnea, 182, 183i
Breast cancer lesions, 320, 321i, 330
Breast dimpling, 322, 323i
Breast engorgement, 328, 329i
Breast lesions, identifying locations of, 314, 315i
Breast lump evaluation, 316
  flowchart for, 317i
Breasts
  abnormalities in, 322, 323i, 330, 331i
    in male, 330, 331i
  changes in, through life span, 308, 309i
  fibrotic changes in, 326, 327i
  inspecting, 306, 307i
  palpating, 310, 312, 313i
    methods for, 311i
Breath sounds
  adventitious, 186, 187i, 188, 189i
  auscultating for, 172
  classifying, 174
  locations of, 173i
  types of, 174, 175t
Bronchophony, checking for, 176, 177i
Brudzinski's sign, eliciting, 154, 155i
Bulla, 25i

C

Candida albicans infections, 294, 295i
Candidiasis, 96, 97i
Carcinomas, 30, 31i